The Coming Physician Surplus

The Coming Physician Surplus

IN SEARCH OF A POLICY

Edited by

Eli Ginzberg
Miriam Ostow

LandMark Studies
ROWMAN & ALLANHELD
PUBLISHERS

ROWMAN & ALLANHELD

Published in the United States of America in 1984
by Rowman & Allanheld, Publishers
(A division of Littlefield, Adams & Company)
81 Adams Drive, Totowa, New Jersey 07512

Library of Congress Cataloging in Publication Data
Main entry under title:

The Coming physician surplus.

   Based on papers from a conference sponsored by the
Conservation of Human Resources, Columbia University,
June 3-4, 1982.
   Bibliography: p.
   Includes index.
   1. Physicians—United States—Supply and demand—Con-
gresses. 2. Physicians—Supply and demand—Government
policy—United States—Congresses. 3. Medical education—
United States—Congresses. I. Ginzberg, Eli, 1911–
II. Ostow, Miriam. III. Conservation of Human Resources
Project (Columbia University) [DNLM: 1. Physicians—
Supply and distribution—United States—Congresses.
2. Health policy—United States—Congresses. W 21 C733]
RA410.7.C57   1984   331.12'916106952   84-4894
ISBN 0-8476-7364-2

84 85 86 / 10 9 8 7 6 5 4 3 2 1

Printed in the United States of America

Contents

Tables and Figures

Tables

Figures

Preface

On 3–4 June 1982, the Conservation of Human Resources, Columbia University, convened its fourth annual conference to assess developments affecting the future numbers and utilization of physicians in the United States. These conferences have been one component of a continuing research effort originally stimulated by unequivocal signs of a vast and continuing increase in the supply of physicians during the remaining years of this century. The origins and earlier stages of this inquiry were reported in the fall 1981 issue of the *Milbank Memorial Fund Quarterly/Health and Society* (vol. 59, no. 4).

As with the earlier conferences, participants in 1982 were invited from many different sectors of the health care system, including undergraduate medical education, the specialty societies, hospitals, foundations, federal and state governments, insurance, health economics, academic health centers, the AMA, and other groups with an interest in health policy.

Unlike its predecessors, the agenda for the 1982 conference, "The Expanding Physician Supply: Policy Options," was structured about a set of invited papers that were distributed in advance to provide the conferees with a common assessment of recent and prospective developments as a basis for discussion.

These six papers, a few of which have been somewhat revised, form the heart of the present volume. Two additional chapters were written after the conference. Chapter 1, the "Conference Summary," reviews the major themes and viewpoints that emerged during the four sessions of intensive discussion, as perceived by the conference chairman.

The concluding chapter, "Directions for Policy," has also been written by the chairman and incorporates the views of his colleagues at Conservation of Human Resources, Mrs. Miriam Ostow and Edward Brann, M.D. Although informed by the prepared papers and by the conference discussions, responsibility for the assessment of the issues and the proposed strategy for policy rests exclusively with the Conservation staff.

Eli Ginzberg, Director
Conservation of Human Resources
Columbia University

1

Conference Summary
The Expanding Physician Supply:
Policy Options

ELI GINZBERG

The agenda for the 1982 conference, "The Expanding Physician Supply: Policy Options," encompassed three major themes: the future of undergraduate medical education, residency training, and specialization; the changing relations between physicians and hospitals; and new and expanding modes of health care delivery. Initially, the discussion focused on likely developments in the number and types of physicians who will be entering practice in the years ahead; later sessions explored how this substantially increased supply would affect the relations of physicians not only to hospitals, but also to a variety of modes of practice, traditional and innovative, with particular reference to the provision of health care outside of hospitals.

Medical School Enrollments

The conferees did not consider it likely that enrollments would decline in the years immediately ahead. They noted that the ratio of applicants to admissions, which had decreased from a peak of 2.8:1 in 1973–1975 to 2.1:1 in 1981, would recede further during the decade of the 1980s (in light of a prospective reduction of about 15 percent in the college age cohort). It would, however, not sink as low as 1.7:1, the nadir reached in 1960 and 1961.

All of the discussants were concerned that with tuition increasing steeply, especially in the nonstate-supported schools where the average for the top quartile is currently between $10,000 and $12,000, young people from low-income families, which include a disproportionate number of minorities, might be discouraged from choosing medicine as a career. This expectation was supported by the fact that the proportion of black medical students had already receded slightly from its mid-1970s peak of about 6.5 percent.

Among the other important observations that surfaced was the likely resistance of financially pressed medical schools to consider any reduction in enrollments because of the concomitant loss in revenues this would entail, the more so since more than half of their faculty hold tenured positions. Nevertheless, several states and some private universities had amended or were about to amend their personnel system to permit institutions of higher education to discharge tenured faculty if necessitated by their budgetary positions.

Despite the prevailing disinclination to curtail enrollments, a dozen or more medical schools for differing reasons—inadequate quality of the applicant pool, state budgetary strictures, pressure from practicing physicians to limit the number of future competitors—were likely to cut back, and others might actually close in the years ahead.

There was no agreement among the conferees whether the educational debts that would burden more and more medical students upon graduation would prove a major deterrent to the numbers who would seek to enter the profession. Nor was there agreement about the rate at which cumulative debt would increase and whether, conceivably, it might be constrained as more students returned to an earlier pattern of working their way through medical school. It was acknowledged that a responsibility for obligations approaching $100,000 upon graduation from medical school would influence students in their choice of specialty, mode of practice, and location, since they would be under great pressure to dispose of their debts as expeditiously as possible.

In a period of higher tuitions and mounting debts, a continuing shift of students from private to state-supported schools is anticipated, the more so because of the increasing scarcity of student grant and loan funds. A few public schools still maintain tuitions below $1,000, and several others charge only slightly more; hence, not all physicians will be financially burdened at graduation.

The conferees noted that enrollments in U.S. medical schools would not account for the entire future supply of physicians. It is necessary to factor into the estimate the number of foreign medical graduates (FMGs) who will enter the system at the residency level, since a significant proportion of them will remain to practice in the United States. Although the number of FMGs dropped precipitously following the federal health manpower legislation of 1976, the most recent data show a new upward tilt.

Even more important for calculating the future supply are the numbers of USFMGs. It was reported that New York State is well down the road to accrediting one or more offshore schools, which would surely increase the potential supply of new physicians. Morever, these USFMGs, estimated to exceed 2,000 annually, represent a "wild card" in any future move to curtail enrollments in U.S. medical schools. Some students will continue to seek medical training abroad if unable to gain admittance at home, even in a period of declining competition for admission.

One informed observer predicted that by 1990, annual admissions to medical schools in the U.S. would fall 2,000 to 3,000 persons below the present level of approximately 17,000.

Changes in Residencies and Specialization

For a variety of reasons, including the ease of financing graduate medical education through patient reimbursement, the advantages to attending physicians of house staff assistance, the contribution of residents to the improvement of patient care, and the enhancement of institutional prestige that accrues to graduate training programs, the last decades have been characterized by more residency positions than applicants and considerably more than could be filled by graduates of U.S. medical schools. But this imbalance has been changing rapidly as the output of U.S. medical schools has doubled and as demands for the introduction of new training programs and the expansion of existing ones have lessened or evaporated.

For the immediate future, the residency matching program reveals a rough balance between the number of applicants (U.S. graduates) and the number of approved positions. But a different picture emerges if one adds, as one must, the 2,000 to 3,000 applicants from each of two additional pools—FMGs and USFMGs. There is the possibility—and it may soon turn into a reality—that some graduates of U.S. medical schools will be unable to secure a residency in the field of their first choice for the year following completion of undergraduate training.

In the past, a small number of FMGs were relegated to practice in the niches and interstices of the U.S. medical care system. Initially, at least, they were unable to secure residency positions; they treated patients, sometimes legally, often extra legally, in special settings, usually severely underserved areas or institutions. If the balance were to tip so that there were more U.S. graduates than residency positions, this marginal pool for the first time would contain a number of physicians who had completed their undergraduate studies in the U.S.

This is neither a certain nor an inevitable outcome of the forces operating in the residency arena, but it does describe one possible scenario. The conferees noted that with hospital directors of residency training resistant to the reduction, let alone elimination, of programs, a new equilibrium might be reached if those seeking training opportunities would accept positions offering stipends considerably lower than the present norms. One conferee noted that it is conceivable that, in extremis, applicants for residency positions might work gratis or even be willing to pay for the privilege.

There is increasing noise in the residency system. While specialty societies inthe past have been primarily concerned with the quality of accredited training programs, should their membership become seriously concerned about overcrowding in the field, quality criteria might be tempered by numerical considerations. Admittedly, fear of antitrust action will inhibit such actions, but if the market were to deteriorate significantly, the specialty boards would be under duress to reduce future output.

As third-party payers, both insurance and government, become increasingly restive about rising reimbursements, the educational costs of teaching hospitals are attracting closer scrutiny. The conferees believed that in the absence of any realistic alternative, neither insurance nor government would refuse to continue to pay for such costs, but they were likely to look more closely at what they were asked to pay. It was noted that New York State made an effort some years ago to limit Medicaid reimbursement to 90 percent of the costs of residency training, but the courts failed to sustain the Commissioner of Health in his attempt to impose this ceiling.

Several conferees observed that another force with the potential of shrinking the graduate training structure was the option some hospital administrators had begun to employ of substituting non-physician personnel, such as surgical technicians, for residents. Others reported that hospital administrators were finding salaried staff physicians to be cost-effective replacements for residents.

Aside from the new pressures generated by increasing numbers of physicians and constrained hospital finances, the residency structure currently in place may be vulnerable to changes in provider and consumer behavior, as Professor Rosemary Stevens has suggested in her essay on specialization and specialty groups (Chapter 6). The conferees found merit in her formulation that larger networks involving more active roles for the medical schools in the placement of their graduates, closer alignments between training centers and large practice groups,and shorter training cycles offering certificates of competence for practice in newer fields might evolve in parallel with ever-increasing degrees of specialization. If such changes were to occur, the extant residency system could be significantly altered in the years ahead.

In the face of large-scale increases in the number of practicing physicians, one must anticipate that the present competition among specialists in neighboring fields, such as internal medicine and cardiology, or neurology, neurosurgery, and orthopedic surgery, will intensify. To the extent that it does, it may alsohave the effect of attenuating the value that physicians now attach to subspecialist certification. Another development may be a subtle structural shift from organization by formal specialty certification to referral mechanisms. Not only hospitals but freestanding specialist groups will explore how to establish and strengthen their relationships with primary care physicians, who are and will continue to be in a preferred position to refer patients requiring more extensive treatment.

Although there has been relatively little reduction, as yet, in the number of residencies, it should be noted that a decline of about 5 percent did occur in 1979–1980. Further, directors of training programs are not infrequently advised by hospital administrators and trustees to leave positions vacant that have not been filled via the match. Moreover, if the federal government moves, as it threatens, to reduce the size and scope of the Veterans Administration (VA) medical services, a significant reduction in residency training positions in state-supported institutions would ensue. If each of the foregoing were to occur, especially if the large training capacity of the VA were curtailed, the impact on the residency training structure would be substantial and the threat of a shortfall in positions for the graduates of U.S. medical schools could quickly turn into a reality.

Relations of an Increasing Supply of Physicians to Hospitals

The chapters by Professor Karen Davis and Professor Frank Sloan are in general agreement that an increased supply of physicians has, in the past, led to a disproportionate rise in total health care expenditures, not so much by increasing payments to physicians, but rather through greater outlays for hospitalization. To the extent that this relationship continues in the future, the increases in the physician supply will result in much enlarged outlays for health care fueled by the greater utilization and intensity of hospital care.

Many of the conferees questioned the validity of econometric forecasts whose projections for the 1980s assume reasonable stability in the structure of medical service delivery that was operative during the 1960s and 1970s. In the opinion of the critics, the 1980s will see major changes over a broad front, including such developments as the rapid growth of ambulatory care sites and the withdrawal of considerable diagnostic work and minor surgery from the hospital; the continued, possibly accelerated, growth of health maintenance organizations (HMOs) and other types of prepayment plans that would reduce admissions to hospitals; the establishment of entrepreneurial practice arrangements, both nonprofit and for-profit, that would also tend to reduce hospital use; a decline in the number of independent hospitals; and diversification efforts by many hospitals in attempts to strengthen their revenues through transformation from traditional facilities into broad-based community health agencies that will provide the full gamut of inpatient acute care, home care, nursing home care, ambulatory care, hospice care, and still other services. The presence of a growing supply of physicians will facilitate these new departures, since many future graduates will be more receptive to salaried employment than their predecessors, who entered practice in the halcyon years.

The conferees were in less agreement on the effect of an increasing physician supply upon the ease or difficulty experienced by new physicians in gaining hospital privileges. On the one hand, it was recognized that if the current staff faced a stable or diminishing flow of patients requiring inpatient care, they would be inclined to resist enlarging the distribution of admitting privileges. On the other hand, if the beds were not filled, trustees and hospital administrators might pursue an opposite policy of awarding staff privileges to more physicians.

Considerable concern was expressed about some untoward consequences that appear to be linked to the increasing supply of physicians. The point was repeatedly made that in areas where surpluses of physicians are already evident, younger colleagues entering practice are unhappy, disappointed, and disgruntled, a situation with ominous overtones for the quality of care they would be likely to provide.

Another discussant reported the discontent of former chief residents in his region who found that they were unable to establish a practice in the area where they had been trained and where they had expected to locate permanently. These disappointed residents were sufficiently vocal to alert the heads of the residency training programs, the trustees of the teaching hospital, and the trustees of the local community hospitals to the need for tighter area planning and an improved balance between the numbers being trained and the numbers who could be absorbed.

Another serious concern was identified by those who saw the rapid move to ambulatory surgery undermining the peer review system that had been laboriously developed by hospitals to assure quality control over surgical procedures. In the absence of new mechanisms for comparable quality control outside the hospital, the not-infrequent performance of ill-advised surgery by poorly qualified, perhaps unscrupulous, physicians would have to be anticipated.

The conferees recognized that with the diffusion of specialists to outlying areas, referral patterns were shifting and fewer patients were being admitted toteaching centers. In fact, several specialty boards had been concerned about the insufficient numbers and types of patients available to provide appropriate learning opportunities for specific training programs with large complements of residents. A related problem was identified as the "dumping" of patients without insurance coverage into certain tertiary care institutions, especially the principal teaching hospitals of academic health centers. Such dumping imposes a severe financial strain on these institutions.

The members of the conference considered the efforts of many medical schools to increase their resources through the expansion of faculty practice plans to be, at best, a limited remedy for their worsening financial condition.

It was pointed out that the highest potential contributors to such a plan often had the option of changing their mode of practice; that there have been cases when physicians, resentful of the pressures brought on them to maximize their contribution, have resorted to the courts that have upheld their right to resist coercion; and that aggressive practice plans invariably intensify town-gown conflicts with dysfunctional results for the academic health center.

In a tightening financial environment, a growing threat to the well-being of major hospitals is the organization by key staff members of a group practice to offer a range of ancillary services outside the hospital and the performance of an increasing number of surgical procedures in an ambulatory setting. Such developments could greatly weaken the financial viability of institutions already under substantial pressure.

Finally, several discussants pointed to the possibility that as the various residency/specialization/practice arrangements that have been identified materialized, they would exacerbate the rising anxiety and discontent of house staff, who would then engage in even more aggressive organizing efforts to gain greater control over their uncertain future. If such organizing activities succeeded, they would represent one more burden for the major teaching hospitals in a period of constrained finances.

Emerging Policy Issues

In the course of the two days of discussion, a considerable number of policy issues were identified and explored in preliminary fashion, even though none was probed in depth. The more important of these will be noted briefly.

It was observed toward the end of the conference that almost no reference had been made to the federal government and its possible actions to influence the future supply of physicians. All agreed, however, that "no policy" is also policy. Moreover, the final withdrawal of direct funding for medical education is already well underway, and the administration is seeking to contain Medicare and Medicaid reimbursements. This will seriously endanger the financial position of academic health centers by reducing the flow of revenues to their principal teaching hospitals. Dean Stuart Altman saw merit in the federal government's exploring how it might make use of reimbursement to affect the numbers, types, and distribution of the future supply of physicians. Dean Altman believes that reimbursement is a more appropriate mechanism for the federal government than direct regulation of supply.

With respect to future actions by state government, a consensus emerged that in most states decisions about the level of support for medical education and medical students will be subsumed within the broader determinations about higher education. It appears unlikely that legislatures would separate medical education from the rest of the higher educational system that they are committed to finance.

Just what measures state legislators will take, and when, to rein in their outlays for higher education, including medical education, will depend on the intersection of the state's budgetary position and the changing perceptions and priorities of the public. Although revenues are likely to be constrained for years to come, the conferees agreed it is premature to anticipate changes in the public's attitudes toward competing state programs. In the past, state legislators have been liberal in appropriating money for higher education in the face of evident manpower stringencies. Once the public no longer complains about a physician shortage and the medical profession warns about increasing competition, many legislators will be inclined to cut appropriations.

One of the conferees believed that the legislature in his state would not fail to respond to the exhaustion of federal grant and loan support for medical and other health professions students: it would definitely seek to pick up at least part of the slack so medical careers would not be open exclusively to the children of affluent families. But this view of prospective state action was not echoed by others.

There was no clear sense of the direction of state policy with respect to allied health personnel. The rise in the numbers of physicians is putting pressure on state legislators not to broaden the practice acts for non-physician providers. Several of these provider groups, particularly nurses, however, are well organized in certain states and are continuing to lobby for greater autonomy. The outcome of these conflicting forces remains in doubt.

Finally the conferees recognized that, thus far, the American Medical Association (AMA) and most other organized groups of physicians have been disinclined to take the initiative and to recommend restrictive actions to lessen the dislocations that a surplus would create. On the other hand, it was acknowleged that silence on the part of the profession makes it more difficult for the public to reach a judgment about whether a problem is pending and what, if any, public action is needed. At present, the position of the AMA appears tobe to provide reliable data about the numbers, composition, and practice modes of physicians so that all of the interested parties—medical school faculties, specialty societies, individual practitioners, and prospective entrants into medical school—can make their own determinations with respect to preferred lines of action. If and when practicing physicians find that the medical care system has reached a point where much of their professional time is idle, they are likely to urge the leadership to reconsider this nondirective stance.

2

The Growing Physician Surplus: Will It Benefit or Bankrupt the U.S. Health System?

STUART H. ALTMAN

That the number of physicians practicing in the United States has grown rapidly in the last decade and will continue to grow through at least the next twenty years is well known and readily accepted.[1] Beyond this, however, there is much disagreement about whether this growth will benefit or bankrupt the nation's health system. There does appear to be a consensus that matching physician supply with the population's health care requirements has not been achieved by the large-scale government involvement of the past two decades. Indeed, many believe that problems have been exacerbated or even caused by government action or inaction. Nevertheless, some have reached the conclusion that our current problems can be remedied only by the federal government or by the medical profession working under powers given to it by government.[2]

Of course, not everyone shares the view that the federal government is either the primary villain or the preferred savior. In fact, many have argued that there is no problem and that even if there is a physician surplus, the worst remedy would be to increase the role of government or the medical profession.[3]

This chapter will review the history of federal influence upon the supply of physicians and some of the factors that led to government intervention in a labor market it had long avoided. It will then analyze the current debate over the recommendations of the Graduate Medical Education National Advisory Committee (GMENAC) established under congressional mandate to review physician supply issues. Last, it will advance some predictions about the likely future of the physician labor market and an assessment of the need for further governmental involvement.

The writing of this manuscript was greatly facilitated by the extensive research of June Mendelson and Judith Williams.

The Supply of Physicians and the Federal Role

The predominant characteristic of the physician supply today is its size and growth rate compared with just ten years ago: the number of practicing physicians increased more than 37 percent during the 1970s and more than 70 percent between 1960 and the present.[4] This growth in the number of physicians has far outstripped overall population growth, resulting in a substantial increase in the physician-to-population ratio. The current ratio of more than 20 physicians for every 10,000 people is 30 percent higher than that in 1970 and more than 40 percent higher than in 1960.[5] Even more significant is the projection that by 1990 there will be 24 physicians per 10,000 population, representing a further 17 percent increase over today's ratio.[6]

Some debate continues to surround the role of the federal government in generating the growth in physician supply.[7] Certainly, the climate in the early 1960s was ripe for such an expansion, when the number of qualified medical school applicants far exceeded available spaces and there was incontrovertible evidence of substantial shortages in the supply of physicians around the country. The medical education system, however, appeared either unwilling or unable to expand in order to increase output. It has been suggested that in time both private and state schools would have enlarged sufficiently to meet this need without federal assistance, and that this self-initiated expansion would have stopped short of creating a likely physician surplus. In our view, the evidence clearly supports the importance of federal intervention as a prime mover in the unprecedented increase in supply that was to follow.

In 1963, after a decade of debate concerning the need for government to remedy a perceived physician shortage, Congress enacted legislation to provide limited support for the construction and expansion of health professions schools and for student loans.[8] Just two years later Congress extended its appropriations for these programs to include basic and special improvements grants to all health professions schools.[9] And, in 1968, Congress again appropriated additional monies for the training and education of both allied health and physician manpower.[10]

There is little doubt that the availability of federal support significantly quickened the pace of construction of new medical schools.[11] Beginning in the 1920s, the Flexner reforms had reduced the number of existing medical schools and introduced accreditation procedures that made the establishment of a new school difficult and costly. Between 1965 and 1967, funding for medical school construction grew substantially and in 1967–1971 fluctuated between $80 and $100 million annually.[12] Student loans and scholarships also grew in that period, reaching a level of $20 million by 1971. These sums, however, were far exceeded by the rise of institutional support that began quite modestly in 1967. This shift in the mode of federal support for medical schools culminated in the passage of the Comprehensive Health Manpower Training Act of 1971.[13] Following passage of that law, funds earmarked for construction fell almost to zero, and capitation or general institutional support tripled, from $60 million in 1970 to $180 million in 1974.[14]

The net result was that the total number of fully accredited schools which awarded the M.D. degree grew from 87 in 1960 to 123 in 1982.[15] In addition, one fully accredited school offered the first two preclinical years of undergraduate education, and three offered programs with provisional accreditation.

Why did the physician shortage emerge as such an important public issue in the 1960s? A number of forces in this period combined to make the expansion of the supply of physicians a national priority. The era of the 1960s was a period of general social and educational reform, motivated by the desire to improve the position of the disadvantaged in society. The Carnegie Commission on Higher Education, long influential in educational reform, supported greater federal involvement in higher education to ensure equality of opportunity for all young people.[16] Medical education was singled out as most in need of federal support because of the acute shortage of physicians, the high cost of their training, and the public concern over equitable health care. Greater federal aid was necessary, in the Carnegie Commission's view, because the states had little incentive to support the training of physicians who might not remain to practice within their borders.

The reform movement also urged improvements in the availability of health care, and pressed for enactment of the Medicare and Medicaid programs. President John F. Kennedy voiced a popular view in his message to Congress in 1963: " 'Health,' as Emerson said, 'is the first wealth.' "[17] The issue, as Kennedy saw it, was the heightened perception of the efficacy of health care that had been created by federal investment in biomedical research; now, by training more physicians, federal policies would make the benefits of these new medical discoveries available to everyone.

The culmination of this general reform movement was the enactment of the Comprehensive Health Manpower Training Act of 1971.[18] The intent of the bill is evident in the congressional hearings held in the spring of 1971. The failure of the health system to meet national expectations in providing adequate health care was attributed to the physician shortage, which appeared to be worsening despite a decade of federal investment. The capitation proposal, which was the favored strategy for the support of medical education, directly linked federal funding to supply through an enrollment-based formula. Also driving this move toward general institutional support was the financial insolvency of the medical schools. The period of rapidly expanding enrollment had plunged medical schools into financial crisis; schools' costs and revenues were both rising, but costs were rising much faster than revenues. The financial distress of the medical schools during the 1970s was shared by their parent universities and by other graduate training programs. Congress took steps to remedy these various problems, but the lion's share of educational appropriations went to the medical schools.

In reviewing the history of federal involvement, one is struck by the rapidity with which the justification for, and objectives of, federal intervention changed. The 1971 Comprehensive Health Manpower Training Act was the last piece of major legislation shaped by the perception of the 1960s that more providers and more federal support for medical education would improve the level of health in the nation. The national debate that ensued when the time came to renew the Comprehensive Health Manpower Act directly challenged this belief.[19] By 1975 few supported the thesis that the problems of our health care delivery system would be solved simply by expanding the number of new physicians. Instead, concern about geographic inequalities in the supply of physician services and the lack of primary care providers became the rationale for continued federal support of medical education.[20]

The 1971 legislation also had been based on a set of projections that failed to take account of the rapid expansion that was occurring both through the output of U.S. graduates and the immigration of foreign medical graduates (FMGs).[21] Whereas FMGs accounted for 23 percent of the number of newly licensed physicians in the U.S. in 1967, by 1974 they had grown to 40 percent.[22] Encouraged by selective federal immigration policies, this new source of physician manpower, which constituted less than 15 percent of all practicing physicians in 1967, had risen to more than 21 percent in 1978.[23] The supply also was stimulated by a new stream: U.S. citizens who began their medical studies abroad, and then entered the U.S. educational system either in the third or fourth year of medical school or at the residency level.[24]

The policy debate was fueled by a faster-than-predicted acceleration of the physician supply and a growing concern that the increasing number of physicians with advanced specialty training was adding significantly to the rapidly rising costs of medical care. The major issue separating the Ford administration and Congress in the debate over extension of the Health Manpower Training Act was disagreement over the need for continued federal capitation support. The administration initially rejected the notion of any capitation funding, but finally acceded to the argument that some federal monies were needed to persuade medical schools to address the twin problems of medically underserved areas and the imbalance in the specialty distribution of U.S. physicians.

When compromise legislation extending the Health Manpower Training Act was finally passed in 1976, the physician supply was still the explicit issue and the medical school was still the instrument of change. In order to address the geographic under service problem, the 1976 Training Act expanded the National Health Service Corps (NHSC), which had been established in 1972.[25] In 1973 only 372 students were enrolled in the NHSC program, which required one year's service in a designated shortage area for each year of financial support. By 1978–1979, there were 4,552 student enrollees, a number lower still than that desired by members of Congress who had proposed a draft of all graduating physicians to fill positions in underserved areas. In 1980–1981, more than 6 percent of all medical students were receiving NHSC scholarships, a level considered excessive by the Reagan administration, which substantially curtailed the program.

The 1976 legislation failed to deal definitively with the issue of specialty distribution. Acknowledging that there was no further need to increase class size, it stipulated a new condition for the receipt of federal capitation funds: that the proportion of first-year residency positions in the primary care fields (general internal medicine, general pediatrics, and family practice) elected by the graduating class should reach 35 percent by 1978 and 50 percent by 1980. This was an aggregate requirement; if the nation failed to achieve it, then each medical school would be held individually responsible in order to qualify for continuing institutional support. Several bills were introduced containing provisions that exceeded these minimum requirements, but these more extreme regulatory proposals were eliminated from the final compromise legislation.[26]

In retrospect, the 1976 legislation had little influence on specialty distribution. A 1977 survey of residents in training revealed that more than 52 percent of the filled first-year residencies were in primary care fields, more than enough to meet the 1980 goal.[27] However, the attrition rate from first-year primary care residencies was substantial. Although the national average was about 10 percent per year, the rate was far from uniform across schools, with private, research-oriented institutions increasingly emphasizing subspecialty programs. Nearly 70 percent of residents who started out in internal medicine were found to pursue subsequently some kind of subspecialty training.[28] At present, there are nine accredited subspecialties in internal medicine and five in pediatrics.

In fact, the most significant trend in medical education in the postwar decades had been the expansion of the graduate medical education system. While congressional debate focused on the appropriate mechanism for federal support of undergraduate medical training, the graduate system was elaborating longer, more specialized, and more complex training programs. The length of time from entry into medical school to entry into medical practice had been effectively extended from the four or five years required by the most restrictive state licensure regulation, to a seven-, eight-, or even nine-year period. The issues of the need and the financial support for this extended cycle of medical education were barely confronted by federal policy.

Nevertheless, graduate medical education is supported by federal money through a number of direct and indirect mechanisms. Direct sources of support include biomedical research funds and training grants; indirect sources include revenue from third-party payers, both public and private. Today nearly $1 billion of federal funds from the Medicare and Medicaid programs, and at least an equal amount of private health insurance funds, underwrite the graduate medical education system. Nevertheless, as late as 1976 no systematic data existed on which to base projections of future supply and requirements for physicians by specialty. To overcome this fundamental information gap and to explore more general new concerns about the supply of physicians, the Secretary of Health, Education, and Welfare in that year established a top-level advisory committee to study what new federal efforts were needed to address the twin issues of physician supply and specialty distribution.

The GMENAC Report

Creation of the Graduate Medical Education National Advisory Committee (GMENAC) was consistent with a historic pattern of appointing a distinguished commission to issue a report prior to passage of major health manpower legislation. Between 1933 and 1970 seven such groups were convened. It is generally acknowledged that one of the most important legislative initiatives in the health manpower arena, the Health Professions Education Assistance Act of 1963, resulted from the Bane Committee Report of 1959.[29] On the other hand, the Carnegie Commission Report of 1970 influenced the enactment of the Comprehensive Health Manpower Training Act of 1971,[30] and not the National Advisory Commission on Health Manpower that had been convened in 1967.[31]

The GMENAC mandate was, broadly, to advise the Secretary of Health, Education, and Welfare on a number of national health planning issues, including how to avoid an over- or undersupply of physicians. The charge to the committee was, specifically, to study:

1. the number of physicians required to meet the future health care needs of the nation,
2. the most appropriate specialty distribution of these physicians,
3. techniques for achieving a more favorable geographic distribution of physicians,
4. appropriate ways to finance graduate medical education of physicians, and
5. strategies for implementing the committee's recommendations.

Reviewers of the GMENAC report are quick to acknowledge that no previous study approaches the committee's efforts in depth of research, complexity of methodology, or scope of recommendations. No one can fault Dr. Alvin Tarlov, the chairman, or his associates for lack of dedication or for timidity.

Nonetheless, many will criticize the undertaking regardless of its rigor, simply because they do not believe that any such study can accurately predict the future.

Most critics ultimately line up either in the "let the market decide" camp or the "let the professionals decide" camp. While there is considerable appeal in the views of the former, it is hard to support the conclusion that the government should have no role in the training of health professionals when it plays such a critical role in the funding of basic and applied research and is a dominant force in the financing of medical services. It seems equally questionable to adopt the opposite position that government's past importance in the training of physicians requires that it now must completely control the size and composition of the profession.

This basic decision about the role of government should rest on a judgment about the costs and benefits of implementing the recommendations of the GMENAC report, relative to other courses of action, such as relying on the self-correcting forces of the market or returning to minimal government involvement. As an interim step in reaching such a decision, the technical aspects of the report must be critically reviewed, but always with full recognition of the ineluctable difficulties of forecasting and predicting the future.[32] A particular problem is that forecasting is usually considered to be more accurate in the short range; the GMENAC conclusions, however, are based on a ten- to twenty-year forecast.

The recommendations of the committee regarding the first three objectives of this study, determinations of aggregate supply and geographic and specialty distribution, rest on a manpower forecasting framework that includes two basic components: (a) the expected future supply of physician services, based on existing conditions in terms of specialty and geographic area and (b) the expected future need for physician services by specialty and geographic area.

PROBLEMS IN FORECASTING SUPPLY

On a relative basis at least, supply projections are assumed to be more straightforward and less subject to error than need or demand projections. Even here, however, the results of past efforts have been less than reassuring. In a review of the GMENAC report, Uwe Reinhardt outlined the many reasons why there has been a tendency to underestimate future supply.[33] He stated, "One of the main difficulties has been the projection of physician immigration, a trend subject to both economic and political factors. An additional source of uncertainty has been the physicians' decisions on retirement . . . and their choice of professional activity."[34]

A third problem identified by Reinhardt is the failure to account adequately for the growing proportion of women in the physician supply. He cited the conclusion of several studies in the U.S. and elsewhere that "women physicians tend to work fewer hours per week and per year and also tend to see fewer patients per hour than do their male counterparts."[35] Predicting the influence of this factor in the future is further complicated by the changing distribution of work roles between the sexes. If trends toward more equal sharing of childrearing and homemaking tasks and the demands of all workers for more leisure time (the average work week of physicians fell from 51.4 hours in 1970 to 50.3 hours in 1978) persist, the traditional male/female differential may narrow and eventuate in a lower rate for both.[36]

The GMENAC physician supply estimates specified a range for two variables: the size of the U.S. medical school output and the number of FMGs entering U.S. residency programs. These estimates assumed increases in enrollments through the early 1980s in allopathic medical schools and through the late 1980s in osteopathic schools, followed by a leveling off of enrollment in each. It was assumed that FMGs entering U.S. residencies would increase from 3,100 per year in 1979 to 4,100 in 1983.[37] Here, as in other sections of the report, I believe the committee edged toward the high side in both projections.

With increased availability of U.S. medical school graduates, the pressure for hospitals to import foreign-trained residents has clearly been reduced.[38] In addition, the estimates of continued growth in U.S. medical school enrollment fail to take into account the end of governmental incentives for expansion, the drastic reduction in federal construction monies, and the deceleration in appropriations for biomedical research. While most of these cutbacks occurred after the completion of the GMENAC estimates, the trend was discernible as early as 1976. Although a large reduction in medical school enrollments does not seem likely, the least expansive of the four GMENAC supply projections may be closer to reality than the "most likely" Case 2 projections (Figure 2.1). The very fact that GMENAC and other reports forecast a surplus may well result in falling application rates as some students opt for other careers. The rising cost of medical education, a decline in the real incomes of physicians, and the scarcity of practice opportunities in desirable locations will surely reduce the rate of return to medicine as a career.

Given the pressures for deceleration in U.S. medical school enrollments and a reduction in the number of entering FMGs, the more conservative Case 3 estimates are more likely. This model leads to an expected supply in the year 2000 of 589,000 practicing physicians, instead of the 643,000 figure generated by the committee's estimates. If these aggregate estimates are further reduced by 10 percent to adjust for fewer physician working hours, the resulting estimate of full-time equivalent supply approaches 530,000, a figure much closer to 498,000, the number estimated to be required in the year 2000.[39]

Figure 2.1 Aggregate Physician Supply and Requirements Under Four Assumptions: 1978, 1990, 2000

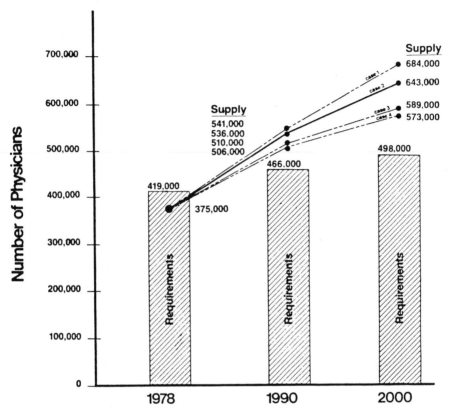

Source: Graduate Medical Education National Advisory Committee, 1980. *Report of the Graduate Medical Education National Advisory Committee to the Secretary, Department of Health and Human Services*. Washington, D.C.: GPO.

PROBLEMS IN FORECASTING REQUIREMENTS

The major dilemma facing forecasters of physician requirements is whether to base their models on expected "need" or "effective demand" for physician services. The term "effective demand" is an economic concept that encompasses several factors: (a) the size and composition of the population; (b) the relative tastes and preferences of that population for the service under consideration; (c) the price or cost of the service, which includes both the monetary price and the time price related to its convenience/inconvenience; (d) the personal income available to absorb those prices; and (e) the ability and willingness of government and the private sector to pay for part of the services (due to the special nature of medical care).

In contrast, "need" is usually defined either in terms of professional standards or of people's perceptions of their health care requirements. Those who support this approach usually do so on three grounds. First, they believe that effective demand is influenced by the existing supply, rather than actual need, and thus produces biased estimates. Second, since the purpose of these projections is to influence private and public policy, they prefer to base them on an estimate of the services that the population should utilize. And third, projections based on demand are extremely difficult, perhaps impossible, to calculate unless it is assumed that existing physician/population ratios and current utilization figures provide an accurate estimate of future demand. But a needs-based estimate can be far off the mark. As Reinhardt comments:

> The needs-based approach makes sense when it is realistic to assume that panels of experts now can develop plausible normative standards for health care utilization 10 to 20 years hence *and* when there is a reasonable hope that the future financing and delivery of health care will be so rearranged as to lead to a faithful translation of normative "need" standards into effective demand. Whether these assumptions are plausible depends, in the first instance, on whether individual consumers 10 to 20 years hence will share the experts' current perceptions of a need for medical intervention. It also depends on the political and economic climate of the future period.[40]

That the political and economic climate can influence the interpretation of professional estimates of need is an important lesson of history. The classic study of professionally determined need, which has served as the foundation for all subsequent estimates, was performed by Lee and Jones in 1933.[41] Using a community medical survey, they determined that 13.5 physicians per 10,000 people were required to provide adequate health care. But they cautioned the reader that although this figure was higher than the existing community ratio of 12.6 physicians per 10,000, it should not be thought to reflect a shortage, since the deficit could easily be compensated by a reorganization of the delivery system. Lee and Jones actively advocated government intervention to provide care for the indigent and to reorganize the health care delivery system into more efficient group practices, rather than simply add to the supply of physicians.[42] As is known, government ultimately did neither.

Given the opportunity for bias in needs-based projections, most economists prefer the demand-based technique. The reason is that effective demand, plus effective supply, determines actual use of services and manpower, rather than professionally determined need.

The GMENAC staff, while indicating that they understood the advantages and disadvantages of both strategies, developed a methodology that, for the most part, relied on the needs-based approach. Calculation of primary care physician requirements was based primarily on professional judgment, since the staff believed that access constraints prevented the market from reflecting the true needs of the population for these services. For the nonprimary care specialties, actual utilization played a more important role, although here, too, adjustments were made using the Delphi group process technique.

A critical component of the forecasting model with respect to aggregate requirements is the expected size and composition of the U.S. population. While the year 2000 is less than twenty years away and most of its population has already been born, substantial changes in the birth rate and the mortality rate can have a significant influence on the demand for physician services.

Unfortunately, official population estimates have been far from accurate in recent years. After several years of maintaining previously calculated fertility rates, the U.S. Bureau of the Census revised downward its future projections of the birth rate. Recently, however, the dramatic drop in these rates has been reversed and there is now a growing sense among demographers that the size of the future population could be greater than currently projected.[43] Because the requirement figures are age-related and because birth and the early years of life generate the need for significant amounts of physician time, a substantial upturn in the birth rate will have an important impact on the requirement estimates of the committee. Nationwide age-adjusted mortality rates have been declining for every age group except youths from 15 to24. Since many observers believe that this group is seriously underserved today, an increase in its size could add significantly to requirements in 1990.[44]

The GMENAC estimates of future requirements also failed to address adequately the needs of another important segment of the population—the elderly. The staff at GMENAC could not examine this issue separately since geriatrics is not a certified specialty. However, they report that the requirements model was adjusted upward for diseases common to the elderly.[45] It is generally agreed that although the elderly are heavy consumers of medical care, the services available to them today are not tailored to fit their needs.[46] In fact, this population, along with the chronically ill, now presents the greatest challenge to the medical system. Although the needs of the elderly are generally met by a complex mixture of medical and social services, the GMENAC projections assume that care for this population will continue to be provided primarily by general internists and family/general practice physicians.[47] Robert Kane and his colleagues, in an attempt to project manpower needs for this age group, concluded that: "In conducting the analysis described in this report, the state of knowledge did not permit us to extrapolate manpower needs on the basis of the abilities of differently trained individuals to bring about the outcomes desired."[48] Clearly, assumptions about the amount and kind of medical care for this population, which is expected to double by the year 2000, combined with the assumption of a declining birth rate, could lead to significant under estimation in the GMENAC projections of the number and kinds of providers needed.

In developing the physician requirement estimates, some attempt was made to factor in the growing use of non-physician providers, such as nurse practitioners and physician's assistants. Using professional panels, estimates were made of the *expected* and *desirable* levels of delegation of care to these non-physician providers by diagnosis. But the use of such physician substitutes is not simply a technical matter: it is a function of the organization of the medical care delivery system, the relative availability of the different provider types, and their relative costs. This availability, in turn, is related to the earning capacity of non-physician providers. The very development of this form of personnel can be traced to the physician shortage crisis of the late 1960s, a situation that will not persist in the future. The committee recognized that without some constraint on their supply, physician's assistants could be used as alternatives to physicians, adding further to the potential of a physician surplus. They, therefore, recommended that "the need to train non-physician health care providers at current levels should be studied in the perspective of the projected oversupply of physicians."[49]

In supporting this recommendation the report states, "At the current rate of training NPs, PAs, and NMWs [nurse practitioners, physician's assistants, and nurse midwives] the supply will double by 1990. The approximated 20,000 non-physician providers in 1978 and 40,000 in 1990 will add further to the surplus capability."[50] While it is likely that physicians will be successful in keeping the demand for physician's assistants from growing, to the extent that the current trend toward greater price-based competition among medical care organizations, such as health maintenance organizations, continues, the demand for these less expensive providers could increase. It seems inconsistent with desirable public policy to prevent this competition from taking place. Premature constraints on the training of either provider type presupposes that we know today what the desirable mix of health professionals will be ten or twenty years hence.

As Table 2.1 indicates, the net result of these various modeling efforts is the prediction that by 1990 the U.S. will have almost 70,000 excess physicians, and by the year 2000 the surplus will approach 145,000.[51] The supply estimates used in these aggregate predictions are those discussed previously as Case 2.

Table 2.1 Aggregate Physician Supply and Requirements: 1978, and Estimates for 1990 and 2000

	1978	1990	2000
Physician supply[a]	374,800	535,750	642,950
Physician requirements[b]	418,550	466,000	498,250
Surplus (shortage)	(43,750)	69,750	144,700

[a]Includes all professionally active physicians (M.D.s and D.O.s) together with 0.35 of all residents in training in the year indicated. The figures for 1990 and 2000 assume that U.S. allopathic medical school first-year enrollment will increase 2.5 percent per year until 1982-1983 for a total increase of 10 percent over the 1978-1979 enrollment of 16,501, and then will remain level at 18,151; that U.S. osteopathic medical school enrollment will increase 4.6 percent per year until 1987-1988 for a total increase of 41 percent over the 1978-1979 number of 1,322, and then will remain level at 1,868; and that FMGs will be added to the residency pool at the rate of 3,100 per year in 1979-1980, increase to 4,100 per year by 1983, and then remain level (Case 2, Figure 2.1).

[b]The requirement figures for 1978 and 2000 are extrapolated from the 1990 calculated requirements on the basis of the population differences in the three years.

Source: Graduate Medical Education National Advisory Committee. 1980. Report of the Graduate Medical Education National Advisory Committee to the Secretary, Department of Health and Human Services. Washington, D.C.: GPO.

There are several plausible alternative assumptions which, had they been used by the committee, would have led to lower supply estimates and larger requirement projections. That, on balance, they are sufficient to produce a state of equilibrium or even of continued shortage is unlikely. Nevertheless, they are of sufficient magnitude to cast doubt on the strength of these surplus estimates and the restrictive policy recommendations that flow from them.

PROBLEMS IN FORECASTING FUTURE SPECIALTY AND
GEOGRAPHIC DISTRIBUTION

Reservations about the technique for projecting future aggregate supply and requirements are minor when compared to the controversy surrounding the GMENAC projections by specialty. At this level few analysts, economists in particular, support the GMENAC conclusions. While the forecasters are to be commended for the complexity of the design and their caution to balance professional judgment with observable data, at the core of their technique is a conceptualization of the labor market and the production process for medical services that is hard to accept. In technical terms, the model relies on a form of fixed coefficients of production. That is, the forecasters mapped meticulously the current practice of medicine and translated their estimates to the future, adjusting only for the relative growth of the different population groups.

Such static assumptions about the production and delivery of medical services conflict with historic experience. Whatever one believes about the future, one fact is certain: it will be different, probably very different, from today. Given the high degree of uncertainty surrounding such fundamental issues as the adequacy of future third-party funding for medical services, the changing structure of the medical care delivery system, and the impact on demand for physician services of future technological innovations, a more conservative approach for projecting demand requirements would have used range estimates for each specialty.

The treatment of each specialty as a separate entity and the resultant aggregate projection of total need implicitly assumes no substitution among specialty groups, an assumption that clearly conflicts with the findings of a 1979 study by The Robert Wood Johnson Foundation. In that study Aiken et al., concluded that specialists did, in fact, provide significant amounts of primary care: one out of five Americans now receives general medical care from a specialist.[52] Faced with projected excess supplies of 190 to 195 percent in the fields of cardiology, endocrinology, neurosurgery, and pulmonary medicine, it seems reasonable to anticipate that some of these specialists will extend their practice to nonspecialty work.

Clearly, we need to understand the implications of this rapidly expanding supply of specialists for the consumer. We know very little about the way consumer preferences for the various types of providers are expressed in the marketplace. In a recent analysis of the demand for physicians in alternative settings, Sloan and Bentkover caution: "Judging from its actions, it is by no means certain that the American public is as convinced as are many policy makers and experts in the health delivery field of the value of services rendered by general family physicians."[53] We know surprisingly little about the changes that will occur in our health delivery system as more specialists and subspecialists enter practice. What are the differences in outcome or effectiveness of care provided by different types of physicians in different practice arrangements? Changes in the organization of medical care delivery from the predominance of solo practice to fee-for-service groups and health maintenance organizations could significantly modify our future requirements for specialists, subspecialists, and physician extenders.

It is clear that the panel charged with reviewing the "methods to improve the geographic distribution of physicians" adopted a different approach from the other groups. This panel seemed to ignore the findings of the physician supply and requirements modeling efforts that pointed to potential physician surpluses and instead concentrated on the problems of the recent past.

In attempting to document the uneven geographic distribution of physicians, the committee concluded that "The systems of data collection necessary for credible geographic manpower planning do not exist."[54] The panel responsible for studying geographic distribution issued thirty-one recommendations, many of them aimed at improving information about geographic variability in the use and supply of physician services and the role of economic incentives in attracting health professionals to underserved areas. The panel also evaluated the efficacy of several government programs that had been designed to assist the geographically underserved, and came out in support of the National Health Service Corps, the Area Health Education Center program, and the use of non-physician providers in shortage areas.[55]

For the most part, the panel failed to consider the possibility that the geographic underservice problems of the past might ultimately be resolved under the pressure of growing surpluses in aggregate supply. While this degree of optimism may not be justified, the report should have explored whether the growth in the supply of physicians during the 1970s has been reflected in shortage areas. It could also have ventured a prediction about the effect upon geographic trends of the accelerated growth anticipated in the 1980s. Surprisingly, not one of the eight topics selected by the panel for review included a time series component or attempted any projections for the future.[56]

THE GMENAC POLICY RECOMMENDATIONS

As mentioned previously, the net result of the modeling efforts was a predicted aggregate surplus of physicians amounting to 69,750 by 1990, and to 144,700 by the year 2000. In terms of physician specialties, the committee estimated that four groups would continue to be in short supply in 1990, eight would be at "near balance" and fifteen in surplus.[57]

These general conclusions led the committee to make the following recommendations:

Aggregate Supply

Recommendation 1.   Allopathic and osteopathic medical schools should reduce entering class size in the aggregate by a minimum of 10 percent by 1984 relative to the 1978–1979 enrollment, or 17 percent relative to the 1980–1981 entering class.

Recommendation 2.   The number of graduates of foreign medical schools entering the U.S. yearly, estimated at 4,100 in 1983, should be severely restricted. If this cannot be accomplished, the undesirable alternative is to decrease further the number of entrants to U.S. medical schools.

Specialty

Recommendation 4.   No specialty or subspecialty should be expected to increase or decrease the number of first-year trainees in residency or fellowship training programs more than 20 percent by 1986 compared to the 1979 figure.

Recommendation 5.   Medical school graduates in the 1980s should be strongly encouraged to enter those specialties where a shortage of physicians is expected or to enter training and practice in general pediatrics, general internal medicine and family practice.[58]

Compared with the requirements that accompanied federal capitation support as legislated in 1971 and 1976, the latter two recommendations in particular appear minimal and nondirective. While the first two recommendations are put in the context of gradual change without specific penalties for failure to make the appropriate adjustments, the committee did state that "Capitation payments to medical schools for the sole purpose of increasing class size or for influencing specialty choice should be discontinued in view of the impending physician surplus."[59]

The committee placed the major responsibility for correcting the potential physician oversupply in the hands of the medical profession and recommended that it should ensure the quality of all graduate medical education programs. It further stated that full funding of graduate training through reimbursement should be provided only to accredited programs where quality control mechanisms are in place.

While the committee stopped far short of recommending a major role for the federal government in the regulation of the supply and distribution of physician services, it did acknowledge that federal funds could be used profitably for: (1) primary care training in family medicine, general internal medicine, and general pediatrics; (2) family practice programs; and (3) renovation and construction of ambulatory care facilities. These recommendations are less directive than some of the proposals that were advocated in the 1970s, such as a requirement that all graduating physicians serve two years in a federally designated location or arbitrary limitation of the number of nonprimary care specialty residencies in order to force more graduates into primary care.[60] Nevertheless, the underlying premise and intent of the GMENAC recommendations are clear: *the current training capacity of U.S. medical schools is excessive and it should be curtailed.* But is a surplus of physicians really a problem?

Is a Surplus Really a Problem?

At the center of the controversy surrounding the GMENAC report is the proposition that beyond a point, ever-increasing supplies of physicians will have negative consequences for our health delivery system. These negative consequences are considered to be of two kinds: an excess number of physicians will generate ever-increasing spending for medical services; and, what is even worse, this increased spending will purchase less and less beneficial medical care, some of which may actually be harmful to the patient's health. Both the increased spending and the decline in the quality of care result from the same factor: the generation of more and more services by physicians in order to maintain their incomes. In economic jargon, the proposition is phrased in terms of the suppliers (physicians) controlling the demand for their services and thus creating a situation where "supply generates its own demand."[61] While few proponents of this thesis believe that the capacity of physicians to expand the demand for their own services is infinite, there has been little effort to ascertain the point in the curve at which this limit is reached.

In terms of national health policy this thesis was clearly articulated by Secretary Joseph Califano in an address to the Association of American Medical Colleges:

> Doctors, after all, make most of the decisions that govern the health care market place. So the chief effect of physician oversupply is dramatically rising costs—without correspondingly dramatic improvements in health status, though certainly some health benefits are taking place.[62]

Some analysts have suggested that given the power of physicians to generate demand for their services, future levels of medical care expenditures can be roughly estimated by simply multiplying the expected number of practitioners by an inflation-adjusted rate of current medical expenditures per physician.

While most analysts would not agree with such an extreme formulation, economists like Robert Evans have supported the hypothesis that physicians can generate enough activity to insulate their work load against supply shifts.[63] He states that "the market for physician services is not self-equilibrating in the usual sense, that price does not serve primarily to balance supply and demand."[64]

The idea that suppliers in a market have such control over the demand for their services is abhorrent to economists. It defies the basic principle underlying classical economic theory that the forces influencing supply and demand decisions are independent of each other. If classical theory has some validity, increases in the supply of physicians would inevitably lead to both a reduction in the price of physician services and an increase in the use of such services. Purists would remind us that price, as stated here, refers to both the monetary price and the time price that accompanies accessibility to the services. It is quite possible, under such a definition, for the monetary price to stay the same or even increase, while the total price (which includes the cost of waiting and travel) declines. In other words, access to medical care is sufficiently improved so that utilization increases.

Basically, what separates economists from most other observers of labor markets is the deeply held belief of the former that such markets are self-correcting and that unless artificial constraints are imposed by government or by the profession, shortages or surpluses will not persist indefinitely. In terms of physician supply such a view suggests that the continued growth of per capita supplies of physicians will lead to reductions in the real incomes of physicians, particularly those in the specialties with the largest growth rates relative to demand. Over time such reductions in real income will lead to a reduction in the supply of physicians or at least in the growth of those specialties with the largest excess supplies.

What is left unsaid in traditional theory is just how long this equilibrating process will take and what will be the final outcome in terms of total spending for medical care. Critical to the final equilibrating figures for physician fees, physician incomes, and total spending for physician services is the question of whether demand for these services can be sustained indefinitely. That is, how many more physician services will consumers use and be willing to pay for? Implicit in Secretary Califano's statement cited earlier is the belief that the demand for physician services, and the physician-generated hospital services as well, are infinitely elastic; i.e., individuals will accept and pay for the ever-expanding supply of services in proportion to their growing availability.

The GMENAC methodology modifies this extreme position by linking the expected increase in demand to the "medical needs" of the population. But here, too, it is assumed that there will be available the financial mechanisms needed to pay for whatever level of demand these need-generated estimates predict. However, with spending for health care already 10 percent of the nation's Gross National Product, and with more and more corporations resisting yearly increases of 15 to 25 percent in their health insurance premiums, this assumption may need to be revised.

In summary, the arguments in favor of limiting the growth of future supply, particularly in the high specialty fields, are based on the view that since doctors make most of the allocative decisions in the health care system and there are few financial constraints to increases in spending for medical care, growth in physician supply will simply translate into growth in health care spending. Further, much of this increased spending will be for medical activities of marginal value in already over-doctored geographic areas.

Counter to this view is the expectation that many positive results can flow from the growth in physician supply. The ready availability of physicians will facilitate the establishment of new health care delivery systems and the recruitment of newly trained physicians by geographic areas in short supply. We also should see a shift away from the popular subspecialties as relative incomes in these fields fall and it becomes more difficult for additional specialists to obtain medical school appointments and hospital privileges.

In my view, the key to which of these two scenarios will prove correct can be found on the demand side of the equation. If we continue to maintain a third-party insurance system that will pay for almost any service prescribed by a physician at a rate controlled by the physician, there is little likelihood that traditional market forces will resurface in this industry to effect a proper balance between the medical needs of the population and the desires of the physician. If, on the other hand, insurance coverage becomes less extensive and new forms of medical care reimbursement that encourage cost-consciousness in consumer and provider behavior are extended, then the worst fears of the "supply creates its own demand" school will not be realized. Accordingly, the controlling factor as to whether the nation will have too many physicians rests not on relative supply, but on the willingness of those who use and pay for physician services to permit the perversion of a potentially beneficial situation.

EMPIRICAL RESULTS

Several recent studies have suggested that even with our present medical reimbursement system, the increasing availability of physician services will produce less than a proportionate increase in demand. Thus, while total spending for medical services will increase, the real incomes of physicians will decline.

Karen Davis has analyzed expenditures for and utilization of medical services in different sections of the U.S. in relation to the per capita availability of physicians.[65] Using 1978 data, she found that in areas of the country with high physician/population ratios, expenditures were higher for all aspects of medical care, but at the same time the net earnings of practitioners in these heavily doctored areas were lower than those of their peers elsewhere.

Interestingly, areas with high physician/population ratios were not found to have lower physician fees. However, while physicians in these areas were able to maintain their fees, they did not succeed in generating proportionate increases in the utilization of their services. Thus, the average incomes of physicians in the highly concentrated areas of Boston and San Francisco lag those of their colleagues in other sections of the country.

The tentative nature of her evidence required Davis to caution against reaching "sweeping policy conclusions" about the desirability or undesirability of an expanding physician supply. But she did suggest that the estimated increases in per capita physician supply could lead to an increase in per capita hospital spending of 12 percent, and a 9 percent increase in expenditures for physician services by 1990. What is likely to elicit the greatest response, at least by physicians, is the projection that per capita physician incomes could decline from $65,000 to between $45,000 and $55,000 in 1978 dollars.[66]

In a less well-known study, two Canadian economists examined the relationship between medical expenditures for the period 1957–1971 in the ten Canadian provinces and the physician/population ratios in those areas.[67] The results of their analysis suggest that expenditures for physician services rise as per capita supplies of physicians increase, but that this rise is not infinite and may be reversible if supplies increase excessively. The study found that as per capita physician supply approached 120 percent of the average for all the provinces studied, the rise in expenditures decelerated and actually declined once it had exceeded 119.2 percent of the average. This limit in the growth curve falls well within the observed increases in Canada and is considerably less than the 28.7 percent rise expected in the U.S. physician/population ratio between 1978 and 1990.

In a less technically sophisticated analysis, Thomas Weil suggests that increasing numbers of physicians in a community can, in time, lead to *reductions* in use of hospital inpatient and outpatient facilities.[68] In an analysis of three case studies he concluded that:

> once there is a minimum "sufficient" number of physicians to meet a service area's needs, adding physicians does not necessarily increase the total volume of patient days in the long run. In fact, based on the suburban areas' experience of having what might be considered a maximum number of physicians and assuming that they have no population growth, adding physicians actually may decrease in-patient utilization over time.[69]

As has been discussed earlier, several federal programs have been designed to address the problem of the shortage of physician services in designated geographic locations. An extensive study by William Schwartz et al. supports the expectation that with the growth in aggregate numbers of physicians, more and more underserved communities will witness an influx of practitioners.[70] Using information from twenty-three states, the authors analyzed the growth of specialty services in small cities and towns from 1960 to 1970 to 1977. For all eight specialties, there was unequivocal growth in the percentage of communities with at least one board-certified specialist.

For example, in communities of 10,000 to 20,000 persons, the percentage with at least one board-certified surgeon rose from 58 to 71 percent between 1960 and 1977; in urology it rose from 9 to 26 percent; and in neurosurgery from 1 to 2 percent.[71] While this unmistakably represents movement in a positive direction, the problem of geographic maldistribution will not disappear overnight. At the same time that the physician/population ratio rose 18.1 percent in urban counties between 1970 and 1976, the corresponding growth in rural counties was only 6.7 percent.[72]

Nevertheless, the more modest rural growth rate should not be dismissed. In the previous decade, while the physician/population ratio increased in urban areas 17.1 percent, it decreased 11.8 percent in rural areas. There seems little doubt that the growth rates in aggregate physician supply expected in the next twenty years will be reflected considerably in rural America. Failure of the GMENAC report to consider this issue is a troubling oversight.

Where Should We Go from Here?

The GMENAC report and particularly its recommendations have continued to be embroiled in controversy since publication in 1980. Critics have variously charged that the report goes too far, that it does not go far enough, and that it reaches its conclusions in the wrong way. The Secretary of Health and Human Services at that time, Patricia Roberts Harris, declined officially to accept the report because she feared that its emphasis on reducing the number of training opportunities for health professionals would disproportionately affect minority students. In a similar vein, others were critical on the grounds that it would reverse the progress that had been made by women in medicine, or that other groups, such as foreign medical graduates, would be denied training opportunities.

Criticism by organized medicine has been of a predictably different nature. Most of these groups have either ignored the report or criticized it vehemently. The stated position of the American Medical Association (AMA) is that a public body such as GMENAC is inappropriate, and that its mandate, if it were in fact necessary, should have been entrusted to the private sector. This view is strongly supported by the American College of Surgeons (ACS), which maintains that if a permanent committee is legislated, it should have no regulatory powers. The AMA and the ACS, as well as the Association of American Medical Colleges (AAMC), disapprove of the

GMENAC study on research criteria as well, claiming that its methodology is incorrect; that we cannot predict the future supply of physicians; and that we cannot judge how many physicians are enough, or how many are too many. Finally, it is the generally held belief of organized medicine that the supply of physicians should be left to the marketplace, the only legitimate regulatory force.

With respect to the marketplace argument, it is self-evident that there is a market for physician services. To acknowledge this does not, however, lead to the necessary conclusion that the forces of the market should be permitted to operate without interference, since the incentives of the market may, in fact, produce socially undesirable results. To assure outcomes that are more beneficial to society, we may want government to intervene and influence the behavior of the market.

While the GMENAC report explicitly rejected government regulation, others could and have adduced its findings to argue that, if the nation does face an excess of physicians in the future and if such an excess will have socially undesirable consequences, it is the responsibility of government to limit the future supply. But does this mean that the only way to control excess utilization of medical services is to reduce the supply of physicians; or that it must be done by curtailing our physician training system? I think not.

Not only do we have a huge institutional investment in medical training, but it is my firm belief that reducing the aggregate supply of physicians by limiting training opportunities will fail to correct the perverse incentives of the existing system. Rather, it is likely to worsen the skewed supply of specialists and urban practitioners and to perpetuate/reinforce spiraling medical care costs.

There are justifiable reasons to reduce capitation support for medical schools, as recommended in the GMENAC report, since this may not be an effective use of federal funds. But this does not imply that we should reduce medical school enrollment. Vast sums of money have been channeled into medical education as a mechanism to remedy past ills, and as a result our medical care system today is greatly improved over that which existed twenty years ago. While we probably spent too much for the cure, few would question the potency of the medicine.

Many benefits can accrue from the ready availability of physicians and abundant educational programs. The growth in training opportunities has allowed more minority students and women to receive a medical education, many of whom are likely to find their way into previously underdoctored areas. Nevertheless, we should not be so naive as to assume that what we have is what we need, or that market forces will militate against a permanent oversupply of physicians. Clearly, current imbalances must be corrected and this will not be accomplished by cutting back on medical education.

The key to solving both the oversupply and the imbalance of physician services lies in altering the prevailing fee-for-service system of payment for physician care and cost-based reimbursement for hospital services. These changes in the reimbursement system should effect a reorganization of the delivery of medical services.

Several promising experiments are now underway in different parts of the country. The federal and state governments have become more aggressive in creating new payment arrangements with the physicians and hospitals that supply most services used by beneficiaries of government entitlement programs. At the federal level, the Secretary of Health and Human Services has initiated a new method of hospital reimbursement under Medicare. The plan is a form of "prospective budgeting" that classifies hospitals and their patient mix on the basis of Diagnosis Related Groupings (DRGs). Hospital payment will no longer be based on retrospectively determined costs. Rather, a predetermined payment schedule based on the cost of treating patients with a given diagnosis will be established, under which all hospitals will receive the same payment for the same service. While there will be regional adjustments and some recognition of the higher costs associated with teaching hospitals, the new system is designed to reward hospitals that are more "efficient" and to penalize those that far exceed the standard rates. The federal system is modeled, in part, upon a program operating in New Jersey. A sample of hospitals in New Jersey have been reimbursed for several years by type of patients treated, rather than by overall costs. The New Jersey system also provides for coverage of free care and bad debts in individual hospitals by a pool of third parties.

Several states, among them California and Arizona, are experimenting with so-called "prudent buyer" or "preferred provider" programs in an attempt to gain control over Medicaid costs. These efforts have also gained the attention of private insurance companies as an approach to the purchase of care for their beneficiaries. This concept requires the covered population to receive their medical care from designated sources, which then are reimbursed according to a pre-established fee schedule. As different as these various strategies are, they share the underlying premise that noncompetitive cost-based reimbursement systems, burdened by detailed governmental regulations, have produced a health care system that is fragmented and highly inefficient. The goal of these experiments is to introduce basic change.

Arizona has implemented a Medicaid program using a preferred provider system. Under the Arizona Health Care Cost Containment System (AHCCCS), each provider organization wishing to participate must demonstrate the capacity to deliver a stipulated benefit package to a Medicaid-eligible population and submit a closed bid indicating the amount to be charged on a prepaid, per capita basis. Medicaid beneficiaries must either agree to receive all of their medical care from an "acceptable" provider of their choice or else be assigned to a group chosen by the state. Under the Arizona plan, patients will not have the freedom to seek care from any provider they wish, nor will the plan pay whatever the provider charges. The number of bids received by the state from provider units willing to participate in the program exceeded expectations, and on 1 October 1982 Arizona initiated its new Title XIX program.

California is in the early stages of implementing its Selected Provider Contract Program. Under this system, Medicaid recipients will be permitted to receive care only from approved providers under contract to the state. Of particular interest to hospitals and to students of rate-setting techniques is Medi-Cal's initial decision to use a flat, all-inclusive per diem rate, rather than a payment system based on the complexity of the patient's treatment in the institution. That is, each hospital must "bid" the per diem amount, inclusive of all ancillary costs, that it will accept for a particular Medicaid population. As with Arizona, the initial response of hospitals has been a willingness, however reluctant, to participate. Students of the health care system agree that had these experiments been attempted five or ten years ago, the provider community would have been unified and strong enough to prevent their implementation. With the growing availability of physicians and the excess supply of hospital beds, these monopoly controls are no longer possible.

A variety of procedures are also being established by large insurance companies and corporations to direct employees and their families to providers willing to deliver services according to a set of medical utilization principles and pre-established fees. In some instances the plan is very simple. It requires every subscriber to "sign up" with an approved primary care (PC) physician. Any procedure approved by the PC physician in any institution will be reimbursed by the insurance company. In other systems, more elaborate medical utilization criteria by diagnosis are being proposed, which must be followed by any provider who wishes to participate in the program. In addition, only designated hospitals will be considered full participants in the plan. If an employee agrees to follow the rules of the "preferred provider" plan, the amount of coinsurance required of him is reduced or eliminated. The level of coinsurance increases if the employee chooses a provider who does not participate in the plan. These plans are particularly intriguing since they attempt to influence the behavior not only of the provider, but also of the individual consumer, who in the traditional insurance system had little incentive to be price-sensitive. Such financing arrangements offer a unique opportunity to assess how increases and decreases in coinsurance affect the individual's utilization of health services.

At the core of all these new types of delivery and financing systems is the attempt to break away from traditional reimbursement methods that permit physicians and hospitals to create an ever-increasing demand for their services. Until recently, most government efforts to effect improvements have consisted of regulatory approaches. While debate raged over the potential consequences of a totally regulated system, the actual incentives that motivate the health system changed little. Now, apparently, we are beginning to see the "market" work.

Whether the reemergence of market forces will lead to socially desirable outcomes or whether these experiments will ever be of sufficient size and scope to have serious impact on a $300 billion industry is still a moot question. But we must not be so cynical that we overlook the importance of what may be the beginning of the most revolutionary change in the health system since the enactment of Medicare and Medicaid in 1965. We should also not be so zealous in our attempt to cut back the physician training system that we rob these experiments of a critical component for their success: the ready availability of new physicians.

Notes

1. Reinhardt, U. 1975. *Physician Productivity and the Demand for Health Manpower: An Economic Analysis.* Cambridge, Ma.: Ballinger; Scheffler, R., Yoder, S., Weisfeld, N., and Ruby, G. 1979. *Physicians and New Health Practitioners: Issues for the 1980's* 1–7. Staff paper. Washington, D.C.: National Academy of Sciences, Institute of Medicine; U.S. Department of Health, Education, and Welfare, Public Health Service, Bureau of Health Manpower. 1980. *Report to the President on the Status of Health Professions Personnel in the United States.* Washington, D.C.: GPO; and Graduate Medical Education National Advisory Committee (GMENAC). 1980. *Report of the Graduate Medical Education National Advisory Committee to the Secretary, Department of Health and Human Services. Volume 1. Summary Report.* Washington, D.C.: GPO.
2. Carnegie Council on Policy Studies in Higher Education. 1976. *Progress and Problems in Medical and Dental Education, Federal Support Versus Federal Control.* San Francisco, Ca.: Jossey-Bass; Comptroller General of the United States, Government Accounting Office. 1978. *Report to the Congress of the United States: Are Enough Physicians of the Right Types Trained in the United States?* (HRD-77). Washington, D.C.: U.S. GPO; and Detsky, A. 1978. *The Economic Foundations of National Health Policy.* Cambridge, Ma.: Ballinger.
3. Demkovich, L. 1981. Assault on Regulators. *National Journal* 14 February:284.
4. U.S. Department of Health, Education, and Welfare, Office of Health Research, Statistics, and Technology. 1980. *Health United States, 1980.* (PHS) 81–1232. Washington, D.C.: GPO.
5. U.S. Department of Health, Education, and Welfare, Office of Health, Research, Statistics, and Technology. 1980.
6. U.S. Department of Health, Education, and Welfare, Office of Health Research, Statistics, and Technology. 1980.
7. Hall, T., and Lindsay, C. 1979. Medical Schools: Producers of What? Sellers to Whom? *Journal of Law and Economics* (Spring):55–80.
8. Public Law 88–129. 1963. The Health Professions Educational Assistance Act.
9. Public Law 89–290. 1965. The Health Professions Educational Assistance Amendments.
10. Public Law 90–490. 1968. The Health Manpower Act. A more complete list of legislation relating to medical education during this period would also include: Public Law 87–415. 1962. Manpower Development and Training Act; Public Law 88–204. 1963. Higher Education Facilities Act; Public Law 88- 497. 1964. Graduate Public Health Training Amendments; Public Law 89–115. 1965. Health Research Facilities Amendments; Public Law 89–239. 1963. Heart Disease, Cancer and Stroke Amendments; Public Law 89–291. 1965. Medical Library Assistance Act.

11. Wallack, S. 1981. Federal Health-Professional Training Programs: Their History and Impact. In *Federal Health Programs, Problems and Prospects,* eds. S. Altman and H. Sapolsky. Lexington, Ma.: D.C. Heath.

12. Association of American Medical Colleges. 1981. *Medical Education: Institutions, Characteristics, and Programs.* Figure 7. Washington, D.C.: Association of American Medical Colleges.

13. Public Law 92-157. 1971. The Comprehensive Health Manpower Act.

14. Association of American Medical Colleges. 1981.

15. *Journal of the American Medical Association.* 1981. Medical Education Issue 246(25):2913. Schools with provisional accreditation but operational in 1981 were Morehouse School of Medicine, Atlanta, Georgia; Oral Roberts University of Medicine, Tulsa, Oklahoma; Universidad Central del Caribe, Escuella de Medicina, Puerto Rico; and East Tennessee State University College of Medicine, Johnson City (the only public school). Mercer University, Macon, Georgia, is in the planning stage.

16. Carnegie Commission on Higher Education. 1968. *Quality and Equality: New Levels of Federal Responsibility for Higher Education.* New York: McGraw-Hill.

17. President John F. Kennedy. 7 February 1963. Health Address to Congress.

18. U.S. Congress, Senate, Subcommittee on Health. 1971. *Hearings Before the Subcommittee on Health of the Committee on Labor and Public Welfare, Health Manpower Legislation,* 1971 1-322. 92nd Congress, First Session. Washington, D.C.: Committee on Labor and Public Welfare.

19. The debate and the views of the multiple interest groups involved in developing the 1976 legislation are clearly presented in Lee, P., and LeRoy, L., eds. 1977. *Deliberation and Compromise, Health Professions Educational Assistance Act of 1976.* Cambridge, Ma.: Ballinger.

20. Lee, P., LeRoy, L., Stalcup, J., and Beck, J. 1976. *Primary Care in a Specialized World.* Cambridge, Ma.: Ballinger.

21. Hansen, W. 1970. An Appraisal of Physician Manpower Projections. *Inquiry* 7(1):102-13.

22. *Journal of the American Medical Association.* 1976. 236(26):2987.

23. *Journal of the American Medical Association.* 1980. 244(25):2814.

24. *Journal of the American Medical Association.* 1980. 2815.

25. The National Health Service Corps was established in 1970 by Public Law 91-623 Emergency Health Personnel Act and became operational in 1972. The scholarship program, Public Law 92-585, was established in 1972 and was extended by the Health Professions Educational Assistance Act, 1976.

26. The Beall Bill (Senate Bill No. 3685) and the Rogers Bill (House Bill No.17084) contained provisions for federal regulation of the number and types of residency training programs. These measures were defeated in the 93rd Congress.

27. Jacoby, I. 1981. Graduate Medical Education, Its Impact on Specialty Distribution. *Journal of the American Medical Association* 245(10):1046-51.

28. Tarlov, A., Weil, P., and Schluter, M. 1979. The Association of Professors of Medicine Task Force on Medical Manpower: National Study of Internal Medicine Manpower III, Subspecialty Fellowship Training. *Annals of Internal Medicine* 91(3):295-300.

29. U.S. Department of Health, Education, and Welfare. 1959. Physicians for a Growing America: Report of the Surgeon General's Consultant Group for Medical Education (known as the Bane Report). Washington, D.C.: GPO. This report attributed the growing need for physicians to the growing number of younger and older age groups in the population.

30. Carnegie Commission on Higher Education. 1970. *Higher Education and the Nation's Health: Policies for Medical and Dental Education.* N.Y.: McGraw-Hill.

31. National Advisory Commission on Health Manpower. 1967. *Report of the National Advisory Commission on Health Manpower. Volume I.* Washington, D.C.: GPO.

32. Rothermel, T. 1982. Forecasting Resurrected: How Forecasting Can Gauge Competitive and Market Forces—As Far as Ten Years Out. *Harvard Business Review* (March-April):139-47; also Harrington, M. 1977. Forecasting Area wide Demand for Health Care Services: A Critical Review of the Major Techniques and their Application. *Inquiry* 16 (September):254-67.

33. Reinhardt, U. 1981. The GMENAC Forecast: An Alternative View. *American Journal of Public Health* 21(10):1149-57.

34. Reinhardt. 1981. 1151.

35. Reinhardt. 1981. 1151.

36. Gaffney, J., and Glandon, G., eds. 1979. *Profiles of Medical Practice.* Monroe, Wi.: American Medical Associaton Center for Health Services Research and Development.

37. Graduate Medical Education National Advisory Committee. 1980. 9.

38. Increases from this source are reduced, but not eliminated. There are no restrictions on entry for Canadian physicians; in 1977, 725 M.D.s from Canada entered the U.S. for training or practice. The Fifth Pathway programs had 2,774 applicants from other FMGs in 1979–1980 and admitted 596 students. *Journal of the American Medical Association.* 1980. 244(25):2815.

39. By the year 2000, about 50 percent of the practicing physicians would have entered the profession after 1975. If we can assume a 20 percent reduction in hours worked for such physicians, the resulting reduction in overall supply equals 10 percent.

40. Reinhardt. 1981. 1150.

41. Lee, R., and Jones, L. 1933. *An Outline of the Fundamentals of Good Medical Care and an Estimate of the Service Required to Supply Adequate Medical Care to the American People.* Chicago, Il.: University of Chicago Press.

42. Committee on the Costs of Medical Care. 1972. *The Final Report of the Committee on the Costs of Medical Care, Medical Care for the American People.* Adopted 31 October 1932. Chicago, Il.: University of Chicago Press.

43. U.S. Department of Health and Human Services, Public Health Services, National Center for Health Statistics. 1979. *Monthly Vital Statistics Report, Annual Summary for the U.S.* Hyattsville, Md.: Public Health Service.

44. Waltron, I., and Eyer, J. 1975. Socioeconomic Causes for the Recent Rise in Death Rates for 15–24 Year Olds. *Social Science and Medicine* 9:383–96.

45. Graduate Medical Education National Advisory Committee. 1980. 24.

46. Kane, R., Solomon, D., Beck, J., Keller, S., and Kane, R. 1980. *Geriatrics in the United States: Manpower Projections and Training Considerations* v. Santa Monica, Ca.: Rand Corporation.

47. Graduate Medical Education National Advisory Committee. 1980. *Summary Report* 24.

48. Kane. 88–89.

49. Graduate Medical Education National Advisory Committee. 1980. *Summary Report* Recommendation 3.

50. Graduate Medical Education National Advisory Committee. 1980. *Summary Report* 25.

51. Graduate Medical Education National Advisory Committee. 1980. *Summary Report* 25.

52. Aiken, L., Lewis, C., Craig, J., Mendenhall, R., Blendon, R., and Rogers, C. 1979. The Contribution of Specialists to the Delivery of Primary Care: A New Perspective. *New England Journal of Medicine* 300(24):1363–69.

53. Sloan, F., and Bentkover, J. 1979. *Access to Ambulatory Care and the U.S. Economy* 127. Lexington, Ma.: D.C. Heath.

54. Graduate Medical Education National Advisory Committee. 1980. *Summary Report* 29.

55. Graduate Medical Education National Advisory Committee. 1980. *Summary Report* Recommendations 19 and 22.

56. Graduate Medical Educational National Advisory Committee. 1980. *Report of the Graduate Medical Education National Advisory Committee to the Secretary, Department of Health and Human Services. Volume III. Geographic Distribution Technical Panel* 7. Washington, D.C.: GPO.

57. The specialties estimated to be in short supply in 1990 were child psychiatry, emergency medicine, preventive medicine, and general psychiatry. The categories near balance: hematology/oncology-internal medicine, dematology, gastroenterology-internal medicine, osteopathic general practice, family practice, general internal medicine, otolaryngology, and general pediatrics and subspecialties. The fifteen categories in surplus: urology, orthopedic surgery, opthalmology, thoracic surgery, infectious diseases—internal medicine, obstetrics-gynecology, plastic surgery, allergy/immunology-internal medicine, general surgery, nephrology-internal medicine, rheumatology-internal medicine, cardiology-internal medicine, endocrinology-internal medicine, neurosurgery, andpulmonary-internal medicine. Graduate Medical Educational National Advisory Committee. 1980.

58. Graduate Medical Education National Advisory Committee. 1980. *Summary Report* 24–28.

59. Graduate Medical Education National Advisory Committee. 1980. *Report of the Graduate Medical Education National Advisory Committee to the Secretary, Department of Health and Human Services. Volume IV. Financing Technical Panel* 23. Washington, D.C.: GPO.

60. The Beall Bill required that medical schools force some percentage of their students to enter a contract to serve in an underserved area prior to admission; the Rogers Bill attempted to improve geographic distribution through the manipulation of residencies to increase the number of residencies in primary care.

61. Sloan, F., and Feldman, R. 1978. Competition Among Physicians. In *Competition in the Health Care Sector, Past, Present, and Future,* ed. N. Greenberg, 48–63. Germantown, Md.: Aspen Systems Corp.

62. Quoted in Davis, K. 1982. Implications of an Expanding Supply of Physicians: Evidence from a Cross-Sectional Analysis. *Johns Hopkins Medical Journal* 150:58.

63. Evans, R. 1974. Supplier Induced Demand: Some Empirical Evidence and Implications. In *The Economics of Health and Medical Care,* ed. M. Perlman, 112–73. New York: Halsted Press.

64. Evans. 1974. 173.

65. Davis. 1982. 55–64.

66. Davis. 1982. 62.

67. Schaafsma, J., and Walsh, W. 1981. The Supply of Canadian Physicians and Per Capita Expenditures for Their Services. *Inquiry* 18(Summer):185–90.

68. Weil, T. 1981. Do More Physicians Generate More Hospital Utilization? *Hospitals* (December 1):70–73.

69. Weil. 1981. 73.

70. Schwartz, W.B., et al. 1980. The Changing Geographic Distribution of Board-Certified Physicians. *New England Journal of Medicine* 303(18): 1032–38.

71. Schwartz. 1980.

72. American Medical Association. 1970–1977. *Annual Reports on the Distribution of Physicians in the U.S.* Chicago, Il.: American Medical Association; Graduate Medical Education National Advisory Committee (GMENAC). 1979. *Interim Report* 91–92; and Calkins, D., and Delbanco, T. 1981. Health Care for the Underserved: The Response of Physicians to a Changing Federal Policy. Proceedings of a symposium on Changing Roles in Serving the Underserved: Public and Private Responsibilities and Interaction, American Health Planning Association, October.

3

Physician Supply and Health Care Costs

KAREN DAVIS

The character and shape of the U.S. health care system promise to change dramatically during the rest of this century. These changes will reflect improving technology, aging of the population, and enhanced standards of living. One of the major forces reshaping the way in which health care is delivered and financed, however, is likely to be the very marked expansion in the supply of physicians projected to occur over this period.

The ramifications of a marked increase in the supply of physicians are not well understood. Little is known about the consequences for access to care, quality of care rendered, and the cost of care. Will an increase in the supply of physicians make care more accessible and affordable, or will an increase in supply lead to unnecessary utilization and higher health care costs? Should policy be directed at halting an expansion in physician supply, redirecting it toward more beneficial uses, or permitting the private market to adjust freely and spontaneously to changes in the numbers of physicians trained?

This chapter attempts to provide some relevant information bearing on these questions by examining the current experience in areas of the United States with widely varying supplies of physicians. The focus of the analysis is the impact on health care costs, although, clearly, information on the consequences of an increase in physician supply for access to care and quality of care is also essential in reaching a judgment about the relative benefits and costs of this expansion.

Background

Traditional economic theory predicts that as the supply of a good or service is increased, price will fall and the quantity of goods sold or services provided will expand. Several econometric studies of the market for physician services, however, would appear to contradict this theory. These studies have found that physician fees tend to be higher, not lower, in areas with more physi-

Karen Davis

cians. Some economists have developed an alternative model of the market
for physician services that argues that physicians have considerable discre-
tion to increase the demand for their services. In areas with a greater supply,
physicians maintain or raise fees, convince patients to return more frequently, perform more tests and procedures, and in general act to achieve a
target level of income.

Other economists have attempted to reconcile a positive association
between physician supply and physician fees with traditional economic
theory. Several explanations have been advanced:

1. An increase in physician supply reduces the travel and waiting times
   patients must spend obtaining services; this reduction in nonmonetary
   costs of care leads to an increase in demand that raises physicians' fees
   sufficiently to overcompensate for the depressing effect generated by an
   increase in supply.

2. Newly trained physicians are attracted to areas of expanding demand;
   such markets may not be in equilibrium and experience an excess
   demand that new physicians meet.

From a cost perspective, these explanations predict that total expenditures
on physician services will be higher in the presence of a greater supply of
physicians.

Few studies have investigated the effects of physician supply on the use of
hospital services, prescription drugs, or services influenced, but not necessarily rendered, by physicians.

Research into the relationship between the number of surgeons and the
volume of surgical procedures has tended to confirm that an enlarged supply
is associated with higher surgery rates. This would suggest that not only are
physician expenditures higher in areas with more physicians, but that hospital expenditures may also be quite sensitive to physician density.

Econometric Estimates of the Impact of Physician Supply on Utilization and Costs

Evidence bearing on how an increase in physician supply over time may
affect utilization of health services and total expenditures for health care
maybe obtained from an examination of variations across geographical areas
at a single point in time. If areas with a very large supply of physicians relative to population experience high utilization rates and high per capita
health expenditures, this may suggest that, over time, an increase in the supply of physicians will elicit similar patterns of utilization and cost elsewhere.

Before turning to a cross-sectional econometric exploration, however,
several caveats are in order:

1. It is difficult to reach normative conclusions about the desirability of any given level of utilization without more disaggregated clinical information. Thus, this investigation can indicate how utilization varies with the supply of physicians but not reach judgments about the need for care that was received. Nor is it possible with this data base to assess the quality of care provided in different geographic areas. While some attempt is made to take into account the need for health care of the population served, measures of need are admittedly crude.
2. Past experience may not be indicative of future behavior. If major shifts in physician supply occur, different patterns may emerge. It should be noted, however, that quite large differences in physician supply are currently found across geographic areas. The Boston health service area, for example, has one physician for every 280 people, compared with one for every 862 people in west central Illinois and one for every 1,786 people in northeast Arkansas.
3. Some caution in attributing causality is in order, pending more sophisticated simultaneous equation estimation and analysis of data over time, as well as across geographic areas.

DATA

The basic data for the analysis are contained in a data file prepared by the U.S. Department of Health and Human Services, Office of the Deputy Assistant Secretary for Planning and Evaluation/Health. Data for 1978 are aggregated from the county level to form average experience of 202 health service areas (HSAs). These areas are defined by the Health Planning and Resources Development Act as health service market areas. Nevertheless, these multi-county units are undoubtedly too large for some primary care services and too small for some specialized services. Adjustments for utilization of services by residents of one area from providers of other areas are made, using data on patient flows from the Medicare program.

Original sources of data include the American Hospital Association for hospital costs and utilization, the American Medical Association for physician supply, the Bureau of the Census for sociodemographic characteristics of the population, the National Center for Health Statistics for health status measures, the Health Care Financing Administration for Medicare program data, and a variety of other sources for miscellaneous information.

Table 3.1 illustrates the wide variation across geographic areas in physician supply, utilization of health care services, and health care costs. The table contrasts the experiences of the Boston HSA, an area with an extremely high physician-to-population density, with that of west central Illinois, a moderately supplied area, and that of northeast Arkansas, an area generally

Table 3.1 Physician Supply, Hospital Expenditures and
           Utilization, and Physician Expenditures and Fees,
           Three Selected Health Service Areas (HSAs), 1978

| | HSA | | | Ratio |
	Boston	West central Illinois	Northeast Arkansas	Boston/ Northeast Arkansas HSA
Physicians per 100,000 population	357	116	56	6.4
Hospital expenses per capita	$477	$289	$165	2.9
Hospital costs per admission	$2,934	$1,273	$670	4.4
Hospital admissions per 100 population	20	19	16	1.3
Length of hospital stay (days)	9.5	8.3	5.7	1.7
Medicare physician reimbursement per beneficiary	$316	$177	$185	1.7
Specialist physician, prevailing charge, routine visit	$15	$10	$9	1.7

Source: Calculated from the 1978 "Health Service Area Data"
         file maintained by U.S. Department of Health and
         Human Services, Office of the Assistant Secretary for
         Planning and Evaluation/Health.

considered to be medically underserved. As shown, Boston has six times as
many physicians per capita as does northeast Arkansas, with much higher
costs per hospital admission. Hospital admission rates and length of hospital
stay are 25 and 70 percent higher, respectively, in Boston than in northeast
Arkansas. Prevailing charges of specialists for a routine visit are 70 percent
higher in Boston than in northeast Arkansas, and Medicare physician payments per beneficiary are also 70 percent higher.

MODEL FOR HOSPITAL SERVICES

While physician supply may be an important determinant of health care cost and utilization, it is clear that other factors also play a role. Sorting out the independent contribution of physician supply requires the development and estimation of a model that incorporates all important determinants.

In traditional economic analysis the average cost of hospital care, like any cost function, varies with input prices, the quantity of care produced, and the quality or complexity of care. That is, hospital costs per admission are expected to be higher in areas where wage rates are higher. If economies of scale exist, average hospital costs will decline with the number of hospital admissions.

Utilization of hospital services in traditional analysis is treated as a demand function and is expected to be lower in areas where the cost of care is higher and where health is better. Ability to pay for hospital care, measured by income or insurance, is expected to increase utilization.

Added to the classic economic model is the hypothesis that a greater availability of physicians will both shift the cost of providing care and induce a greater demand for hospital services. In deference to Roemer's law that hospital bed supply creates its own demand, it is customary to include hospital bed supply as a possible determinant of utilization as well.

HOSPITAL ECONOMETRIC FINDINGS

Econometric estimates of hospital costs and utilization are presented in Table 3.2. As indicated, physician supply is positively associated with hospital costs per admission, admissions per capita, and length of hospital stay. That is, in areas with more physicians, hospital costs per patient are higher, more patients are admitted to the hospital, and patients stay in the hospital longer. The cost of hospital care per patient admitted is especially sensitive to physician supply. An area with twice as many physicians per capita can be expected to have costs per admission that are 32 percent higher than the less amply supplied area, 7 percent more hospital admissions per capita, and hospital stays that are 19 percent longer. Cumulatively, hospital costs per capita will be 58 percent higher in an area with twice as many physicians.

The volume of surgery is also positively associated with the supply of surgeons. An area with twice as many surgeons per capita would be expected to have 23 percent more surgical operations per capita than the less supplied area. This result confirms the findings of numerous other studies linking the supply of surgeons with increased surgery.

If a higher proportion of area physicians are specialists, hospital admission rates are higher. That is, if two geographic areas have the same number of physicians per capita but one area has twice as many specialists, the latter will have 21 percent more hospital admissions per capita.

Table 3.2   Log Linear Econometric Estimates of Hospital
            Expenditures and Utilization, 1978

Independent variable	Hospital costs per admission	Admissions per 100 population	Length of hospital stay	Surgical operations per 100 population
Physician supply	.32 [8.18]	.07 [2.62]	.19 [5.38]	-- --
Surgeon supply	-- --	-- --	-- --	.23 [11.33]
Percent specialists	-- --	.21 [3.04]	.09 [1.08]	-- --
Hospital wage rates	.55 [5.81]	-- --	-- --	-- --
Percent no insurance	-- --	-- --	-.22 [-10.14]	-.05[a] [-2.04]
Medicare case mix	.09 [2.92]	-- --	-- --	-- --
Infant mortality	-- --	.21 [5.20]	-- --	-- --
Percent teaching hospital	.08 [5.09]	-- --	-- --	-- --
Admissions per 100 population	-.13[a] [-2.40]	-- --	-- --	-- --
Cost per admission	-- --	-.24 [-6.71]	-- --	-- --
Cost per patient day	-- --	-- --	-.30 [-6.05]	-- --
Beds per 1,000 population	-- --	.66 [27.92]	.14 [3.85]	.58 [16.20]
R^2	.77	.85	.61	.67

[a]Indicates significance at P=.05.

Note: t-scores are shown in brackets.

Source: Author's calculations.

Results for other determinants of hospital costs and utilization also corro-
borate previous studies. Wage rates are strongly associated with higher costs.
Hospitals in areas where wage rates are twice as high will have hospital costs
55 percent higher than hospitals in the lower wage rate area. This is to be

expected, inasmuch as labor costs represent about 55 percent of all hospital costs.

Measures included in the model to control for quality of care and differences in complexity of cases also have the expected results. Hospital costs per admission are higher in areas with a more complex Medicare case mix (measured by percentage of patients with multiple diagnoses). Costs are also significantly higher in areas with a higher proportion of teaching hospitals, presumably as a reflection of the higher quality of care provided in such institutions. Hospital costs per admission are slightly lower in areas with a higher admission rate per population. This may reflect economies of scale in the provision of care, or it may suggest that the average complexity of patient diagnoses is less in areas where more patients are admitted.

Utilization of hospital services is negatively related to the cost of care. In areas where hospital costs are twice as high, 24 percent fewer patients are admitted. This price elasticity is quite similar to that found in other econometric studies. Similarly, the length of stay in hospitals is sensitive to price. Areas where hospital costs are twice as high will have 30 percent shorter hospital stays. The greater the proportion of the area population with no insurance, the shorter will be the hospital stays.

Income did not prove to be a significant explanator of utilization, perhaps reflecting the fact that a higher income population, while more able to afford care, is also likely to be healthier. Available measures of health status, such as infant mortality, although significant in explaining admission rates, may not capture all variation in health status across geographic areas.

Roemer's law appears to hold, in that areas with a greater concentration of hospital beds also have higher utilization rates. This bed supply effect is quite strong. Other things being equal, an area with twice as many hospital beds per capita will have 66 percent more hospital admissions and 14 percent longer stays, or a total of 80 percent more patient days per capita. Surgical operations are also sensitive to bed supply. An area with twice as many hospital beds can be expected to have 58 percent more surgical operations per capita.

PHYSICIANS' SERVICES

Analysis of physician expenditures and utilization is hampered by the limited availability of data on a small-area basis. The best source of data comes from the experience of the elderly under the Medicare program. Table 3.3 presents log linear econometric estimates of Medicare reimbursement for physician services per beneficiary and prevailing charges of general practitioners and specialists for a routine office visit.

As shown, Medicare physician expenditures per Medicare beneficiary are positively associated with physician supply. For example, an area with twice

Table 3.3 <u>Log Linear Econometric Estimates of Physician</u>
           <u>Expenditures and Fees, 1978</u>

Independent variable	Medicare physician reimbursement per beneficiary	Prevailing charge per routine visit	
		GP	Specialist
Physician supply	.19 [4.06]	--	--
GP supply	--	-.07[a] [-1.98]	--
Specialist supply	--		.06 [2.86]
Income	.52 [5.13]	.36 [5.38]	.19 [2.67]
Wage rates	.53 [4.71]	.46 [5.82]	.54 [6.49]
R^2	.57	.46	.50

[a]Indicates significance at P=.05.

<u>Note</u>: t-scores are shown in brackets.

<u>Source</u>: Author's calculations.

as many physicians per capita could be expected to have 19 percent higher physician expenditures per person covered by Medicare. High expenditures would appear to occur primarily because Medicare beneficiaries in areas of high physician supply receive more services. Charges of general practitioners are lower where there are relatively more GPs, but the relationship is only marginally significant. Specialist charges, on the other hand, are significantly higher in areas with a greater concentration of specialists. Thus, at least within the range of physician supply observed across health service areas, a greater supply of physicians does not result in lower fees, and in the case of specialists results in somewhat higher fees. As expected, prevailing charges and Medicare physician expenditures tend to be higher in high wage rate areas, suggesting that physician fees are sensitive to practice costs. Fees also tend to be higher in areas where per capita incomes are higher, suggesting that ability to pay influences the level of fees.

The implications of physician supply for physicians' incomes are harder to explore, since physician incomes are not published on a small-area basis.

Data from the American Medical Association on census divisions, however, are instructive. As shown in Table 3.4, physician supply varies from 110 physicians per 100,000 population in the east south central region of the U.S., to 183 physicians per 100,000 in New England.

Some interesting patterns are apparent even at this level of aggregation. Physicians in regions well supplied with doctors see fewer patients per week. For example, there are 66 percent more physicians per capita in New England than in the east south central region, and the former see almost 40 percent fewer patients per week.

As was found with the Medicare data, competition for patients does not appear to have the effect of lowering physician fees. Fees run 20 to 30 percent higher in New England than in the east south central region. An appendectomy in the Pacific region, also a relatively well-supplied area, costs more than $500, compared with less than $300 in the east south central region.

Striking differences in practice expenses and physician net income do exist across regions. Areas with more physicians tend to have lower practice expenses per physician, in large part because such physicians hire fewer ancillary personnel. Even with lower practice costs, however, physicians in well-supplied areas have substantially lower net incomes. For example, physicians in New England earn on average only 69 percent of net incomes earned by physicians in the east south central region. That is, while physicians may be able to maintain fees in well-supplied areas, increases in utilization of services cannot be counted upon to assure achieving comparable incomes per physician.

PROJECTIONS TO 1990

The econometric results obtained from the cross-sectional data permit estimates of the impact of increases in physician supply over time on health care costs and utilization. Since the estimates shown in Tables 3.2 and 3.3 are in log linear form, the coefficients are elasticities (i.e., the percent change in the dependent variable caused by a percent change in the independent variable).

GMENAC estimates that over the period 1978 to 1990, the aggregate supply of physicians will increase by 43 percent and the per capita supply by 28 percent. The estimates in Table 3.2 predict that a 28 percent increase in physicians per capita will lead to a 16 percent increase in hospital expenditures per capita and a 3 percent increase in physician expenditures per capita. It is clear from these estimates that the major implications for costs are not the direct outlays for an increased number of physicians, but rather the indirect costs of services generated by physicians in the hospital setting.

These increased health expenditures can be expressed in dollar terms. In 1980 dollars and population, an increase in physicians per capita of 28 percent would increase hospital expenditures by $16 billion, and physician

Table 3.4 Physician Supply and Characteristics of Physician Practice, by Census Division, 1978-1979

Census division	Physicians per 100,000 population	Patient visits per MD per week	Fee			Average	
			Initial visit	Follow-up visit	Appen-dectomy	Professional expense	Net income
New England	183	97.8	$31	$21	$348	$31,100	$54,900
Middle Atlantic	176	118.1	33	21	391	39,600	59,100
Pacific	174	106.1	35	22	503	53,100	64,900
South Atlantic	143	125.6	31	20	383	45,800	64,900
Mountain	138	122.8	27	18	396	48,700	61,800
East North Central	132	132.8	27	17	321	45,800	69,900
West North Central	127	135.9	23	15	298	47,400	70,200
West South Central	120	129.3	30	19	342	52,400	70,900
East South Central	110	158.5	26	16	298	53,100	79,700
Ratio New England to East South Central	1.66	.62	1.19	1.31	1.17	.59	.69

Source: American Medical Association. 1980. Profile of Medical Practice, 1980. Chicago: American Medical Association.

expenditures by $2 billion, together $18 billion out of total hospital and physician expenditures of $147 billion in 1980.

In 1990 dollars and population, the increase in physicians per capita will result in an increase of $54 billion in hospital expenditures and of $5 billion in physician expenditures for a total of $59 billion, out of total hospital and physician expenditures of $463 billion projected to occur in 1990.

Admittedly, these estimates are rough approximations. If in the future more physicians enter salaried practice or work for organizations paid on a capitation basis, some of the increases in hospital expenditures may not be realized. On the other hand, to the extent that an increasing proportion of physicians subspecialize, costs may be even higher. Costs of prescription drugs, nursing home care, and other services may also rise with an expanding supply of physicians. Changing technology, insurance coverage, or reimbursement methods could also radically affect these projections.

Speculation about future physician incomes is even more problematic, given the absence of disaggregated data on which to sort out the independent contribution of a number of important determinants. Yet the very marked difference in physician net incomes across geographic areas today suggests that a major expansion in physician supply may have a depressing effect on physician income. If current patterns across areas are extrapolated into projected future supply, physician net incomes could drop from $65,000 in 1978 to around $55,000 in 1990 (in 1978 dollars). While this analysis is too elementary to warrant much confidence in this estimate, it does suggest that real incomes of physicians will continue to decline in the 1980s as they have in the 1970s.

It is unclear without more disaggregated data whether lower physician net incomes in well-supplied areas are the result of lower earnings by newly trained physicians, while older physicians maintain their incomes, or whether all physicians are affected. Similarly, reductions may be across the board or limited to certain specialties. The more detailed analysis that could be conducted with AMA survey data would be informative.

Conclusion

Empirical results based upon current experience in the U.S. suggests that an increase in the supply of physicians over the 1980s will have a significant impact on increasing health care costs, especially hospital costs. It may be that an increased supply will bring with it benefits that outweigh those costs. For example, access to care for the disadvantaged may be improved or the quality of care may be enhanced. On the other hand, the increased supply may bring few, if any, benefits, and result in increased utilization of services of a marginally beneficial or even harmful nature. Further research on the

effect of increased supply on access and quality would be an important
undertaking.

In any event, the supply of physicians for the 1990s is already in the pipe-
line. Policy efforts may most appropriately be directed to designing incentives to ensure that the increased supply yields the greatest benefits. This
might include incentives for physicians to locate in rural and inner-city
areas, or to expand services to population groups with unmet needs. Expansion of services to homebound elderly, for example, might improve the quality of life for the aging and enable many to avoid expensive institutionaliza-
tion in nursing homes.

Promising research avenues include:

1. Exploration of the impact of an expanding supply on access to care.
2. Investigation into the effects of physician supply upon the nature of
   medical practice. What do physicians do differently when they are in
   relative abundance, and is that good or bad for patients?
3. Case studies of U.S. cities or international experience to provide deeper
   insight into the dynamics of change in the medical market.
4. Analyses on time-series data or other cross-sectional bases to increase
   confidence in the results of the analysis presented here, which is based
   on aggregate data from a single point in time.

4

Implications of the Expanding Physician Supply for Medical Schools and Medical Students

AUGUST G. SWANSON, M.D.

The implications of the expanding physician supply for medical schools and medical students must be considered in the context of the rapid expansion of medical education in the United States during the past two decades. This growth was accompanied by a change in the societal role of medical schools as well—a change that is exemplified by the appellation "academic medical center" that has replaced "medical school." These institutions now have faculties responsible for an undergraduate medical education program, multiple graduate medical education programs, sponsored biomedical research programs, sponsored clinical services programs, and an expanding load of clinical services to the citizens in their locality, region, and the nation. The increase in the physician supply may affect the centers in multiple ways; in addition, a change in one category of program will invariably affect others in these institutions. The interaction between an increasing supply of physicians and various sectors of the health care delivery system will have further ramifications for the complex institutions called academic medical centers.

The Era of Expansion

Between 1959 and 1979 the number of medical schools in the U.S. increased from 87 to 126 (see Appendix 4A). The total first-year class increased from 8,173 to 16,930, and the size of the average entering class rose from 94 to 134 (Table 4.1). During the 1960s growth resulted principally from the addition of 23 new schools. During the 1970s, when only 16 new schools were established, the expansion of older schools was a major contribution to the increased capacity.

Table 4.1   *The Era of Expansion, 1959–1979*

	1959	1969	1979
Number of schools	87	110	126
First-year class	8,173	10,422	16,930
Average class/school	94	94	134

Source: Association of American Medical Colleges.

APPLICANTS AND MATRICULANTS

The enlargement of capacity was accompanied by three significant changes in applicants and matriculants (Tables 4.2 and 4.3). First, the number of applicants per position increased dramatically—from a nadir of 1.7 in 1960 (the lowest recorded since World War II) to a peak of 2.8 in 1973, 1974, and 1975 when more than 42,000 candidates applied each year. Second, the proportion of females applying and matriculating increased from 11 percent and 9 percent, respectively, in 1965, to 30 percent and 29 percent in 1980. This shift occurred almost entirely during the 1970s. Third, the number of applicants from disadvantaged minority groups began to increase in the early 1970s, rose to about 3,500 per year, and plateaued. The proportion of minority matriculants has stabilized at between 8 percent and 9 percent since 1975. These changes in applicants and matriculants have generally been considered to be positive and desirable.

FACULTY AND REVENUE

The doubling of class size was accompanied by a fourfold increase in the full-time faculties (Table 4.4). This expansion was heavily concentrated in clinical departments (fivefold), as compared to preclinical departments, where the faculty increased threefold.

That the expansion of faculties was only marginally related to the expansion of undergraduate medical education programs is shown in Tables 4.5–4.7. In current dollars, unrestricted revenues increased by a factor of 15 (5.6 in 1960 dollars); restricted revenues for sponsored programs increased by a factor of 11 (3.8 in 1960 dollars). These increases in revenue were accompanied by shifts in sources. The proportion of revenue from state and local governments remained constant, while tuition and endowments declined as

Table 4.2   Applicants and New Entrants, Selected Years

	1965		1970		1975		1980	
	Number	%	Number	%	Number	%	Number	%
Applicants								
Male	17,027	89	22,253	89	32,728	77	25,436	70
Female	1,676	11	2,734	11	9,575	23	10,664	30
Total	18,703	100	24,987	100	42,303	100	36,100	100
New entrants								
Male	7,755	91	9,941	89	11,398	76	11,832	71
Female	799	9	1,228	11	3,512	24	4,758	29
Total	8,554	100	11,169	100	14,910	100	16,590	100
Ratio of applicants/ new entrants	2.2		2.2		2.8		2.2	

Source: Association of American Medical Colleges.

Table 4.3   Disadvantaged Minority Applicants and New Entrants, 1975, 1980

	1975				1980			
	Applicants		Entrants		Applicants		Entrants	
	Number	%	Number	%	Number	%	Number	%
Black American	2,288	5.0	945	6.0	2,594	7.0	1,057	6.0
Native American	132	0.3	57	0.4	147	0.4	62	0.4
Mexican American	427	1.0	220	1.0	449	1.0	191	1.0
Mainland Puerto Rican	202	0.4	86	0.6	191	0.5	102	0.6
Total	3,049	7.0%	1,308	9.0%	3,381	9.0%	1,412	8.0%

Note: Percentage refers to total applicants and new entrants respectively.

Source: Association of American Medical Colleges.

Table 4.4   *Number of Full-Time Faculty, 1960, 1970, 1979*

	1960	1970	1979
Preclinical	4,023	8,283	13,039
Clinical	7,201	19,256	36,566
Total	11,224	27,539	49,605
Average/school	129	250	393

Source: Association of American Medical Colleges.

revenue sources. Restricted revenue for research also declined in proportion, while revenue from contracts for services (predominantly medical) increased.

The most striking shift in revenue is the total amount derived from medical services (Table 4.7). In 1960 the schools derived only 17 percent of their operating budget from income received for medical services by the faculty; that source now accounts for 40 percent. One observer has noted that medical schools are becoming appendages of their teaching hospitals. This dependence on income from medical services to support institutional programs may be a source of conflict as the supply of physicians expands.

The Present

In the fall of 1981, 16,644 students matriculated in 126 accredited medical schools (Table 4.8). The largest entering classes were at the University of Illinois (325) and the University of Indiana (305); the smallest were at Marshall University in Huntington, West Virginia (36) and Texas A & M (32). The state with the largest number of entering students in public medical schools was Texas (944), and the state with the largest entering class in private medical schools was New York (1,102). Based on past attrition experience, the yield of graduates from the 1981 entering class is expected to be between 15,800 and 16,000. If present trends in career plans continue, 95 percent of these graduates will take three or more years of graduate medical education and will proportionately seek certification in the various specialties and subspecialties as shown in Table 4.9.

Many of these students will graduate with high levels of debt. The proportion of graduates with debts has ranged around 76 percent during the past decade. Average indebtedness has risen from $5,500 in 1970 to $19,700 in

Table 4.5 Sources of Unrestricted Revenues for General
           Operations, 1960, 1970, 1979

	1960	1970	1979
	(percentage distribution)		
State, local government	32%	37%	35%
Indirect costs	9	13	10
Medical service plans	6	15	20
Tuition, fees	13	8	9
Endowment, gifts	13	7	4
Other	27	20	22
Total dollars (millions)	$214	$780	$3,316

Source: Association of American Medical Colleges.

Table 4.6 Sources of Restricted Revenues for Sponsored
           Programs, 1960, 1970, 1979

	1960	1970	1979
	(percentage distribution)		
Research	76%	52%	53%
Training	22	24	23
Services	3	25	25
Total dollars (millions)	$222	$933	$2,386

Source: Association of American Medical Colleges.

Table 4.7 Revenues from Medical Services, 1960, 1970, 1979
           (millions of dollars)

	1960	1970	1979
Faculty practice plans	$ 13	$115	$670
Hospitals, clinics	22	58	380
Medical service contracts	5	172	448
Total	$ 40	$345	$1,498
Percentage of unrestricted revenue for general operations	17%	34%	40%

Source: Association of American Medical Colleges.

Table 4.8 Entering Class by State and Institution, 1981
Public Institutions

Alabama	214	Missouri	204
Alabama, Birmingham	150	Mo.-Columbia	110
South Alabama*	64	Mo.-Kansas City*	94
Arizona*	88	Nebraska	153
Arkansas	135	U. of Nebraska	153
California	606	Nevada*	48
Ca.-San Francisco	146	New Jersey	300
Ca.-Los Angeles	139	UCMD-N.J.	170
Ca.-Irvine*	96	UCMD-Rutgers*	130
Ca.-San Diego*	125	New Mexico*	73
Ca.-Davis*	100	New York	576
Colorado	118	SUNY-Buffalo	135
Connecticut	80	SUNY-Downstate	220
U. of Conn.*	80	SUNY-Upstate	145
Florida	180	SUNY-Stony Brook*	76
Florida	84	North Carolina	212
South Florida*	96	North Carolina	160
Georgia	180	East Carolina*	52
Med. Coll. of Ga.	180	North Dakota	68
Hawaii*	67	Ohio	767
Illinois	397	Cincinnati	192
U. of Illinois	325	Ohio State	233
South Illinois*	72	Ohio at Toledo*	150
Indiana	305	Wright State*	100
Iowa	175	Northeastern Ohio*	92
Kansas	200	Oklahoma	176
Kentucky	243	U. of Oklahoma	176
Kentucky	108	Oregon	115
Louisville	135	Pennsylvania	98
Louisiana	283	Penn. State*	98
LSU-New Orleans	180	South Carolina	216
LSU-Shreveport*	103	Med. U. of S.C.	165
Maryland	331	U. of S.C.-Columbia*	51
Maryland	175	South Dakota	65
Uniformed Services*	156	Tennessee	252
Massachusetts	102	Tennessee	204
U. of Mass.	102	East Tennessee*	48
Michigan	643	Texas	944
U. of Michigan	287	Texas-San Antonio*	202
Wayne State	251	Texas-Southwestern	205
Mich. State*	105	Texas-Galveston	203
Minnesota	286	Texas-Houston*	202
Minn.-Minneapolis	238	Texas Tech*	100
Minn.-Duluth*	48	Texas A & M*	32
Mississippi	150	Utah	100

Vermont	93	West Virginia	88
Virginia	307	Marshall*	36
U. of Virginia	139	Wisconsin	159
Med. Coll. of Va.	168	U. of Wisconsin	159
Washington	175	Puerto Rico	150
West Virginia	124	U. of Puerto Rico	150

Private Institutions

California	362	New York	1,102
Loma Linda	140	Albany	128
Southern California	136	Columbia	150
Stanford	86	Cornell	102
Connecticut	102	Albert Einstein	179
Yale	102	New York Medical	175
District of Columbia	483	New York University	168
Georgetown	205	Rochester	100
George Washington	150	Mt. Sinai*	100
Howard	128	North Carolina	222
Florida	136	Bowman Gray	108
Miami	136	Duke	114
Georgia	142	Ohio	138
Emory	110	Case Western Reserve	138
Morehouse*	32	Oklahoma	48
Illinois	668	Oral Roberts U.*	48
Chicago Medical	143	Pennsylvania	977
U. of Chic.-Pritzker	104	Hahnemann	180
Loyola-Stritch	130	Jefferson	223
Northwestern	171	U. of Pennsylvania	161
Rush*	120	Pittsburgh	136
Louisiana	148	Temple	177
Tulane	148	Med. Coll. of Penn.	100
Maryland	124	Rhode Island	61
Johns Hopkins	124	Brown*	61
Massachusetts	447	Tennessee	216
Boston University	135	Meharry	112
Harvard	166	Vanderbilt	104
Tufts	146	Texas	168
Minnesota	40	Baylor	168
Mayo*	40	Virginia	96
Missouri	278	Eastern Virginia*	96
St. Louis	156	Wisconsin	200
Wash. U.-St. Louis	122	Med. Coll. of Wisc.	200
Nebraska	108	Puerto Rico	138
Creighton	108	Ponce Sch. of Med.*	60
New Hampshire	85	U. Del Caribe*	78
Dartmouth	85		

*Organized since 1960.

Table 4.9 Specialty or Subspecialty Choice of 8,809 Medical School Graduates, 1981

Specialty	Number	%	Specialty	Number	%
Allergy, immunology	19	0.2	Otolaryngology	174	2.0
Anesthesiology	342	3.9	Pathology	222	2.5
Critical care	28	0.3	Pediatrics	644	7.3
Colon, rectal surgery	4	0.0	Cardiology	33	0.4
Dermatology	107	1.2	Critical care	11	0.1
Emergency medicine	230	2.6	Endocrinology	17	0.2
Family practice	1,528	17.3	Hematology-oncology	34	0.4
Internal medicine	1,118	12.7	Nephrology	9	0.1
Cardiovascular disease	151	1.7	Neonatal-perinatal medicine	25	0.3
Critical care	28	0.3	Physical medicine, rehabilitation	50	0.6
Endocrinology, metabolism	47	0.5	Plastic surgery	113	1.3
Gastroenterology	65	0.7	Preventive medicine	16	0.2
Hematology	40	0.5	Psychiatry	348	4.0
Infectious disease	49	0.6	Child psychiatry	72	0.8
Medical oncology	64	0.7	Neurology	108	1.2
Nephrology	31	0.4	Child neurology	14	0.2
Pulmonary disease	21	0.2	Radiology	22	0.2
Rheumatology	23	0.3	Diagnostic radiology	410	4.7
Neurological surgery	111	1.3	Therapeutic radiology	31	0.4
Nuclear medicine	8	0.1	Surgery	556	6.3
Obstetrics, gynecology	552	6.3	Critical care	23	0.3
Gynecologic oncology	35	0.4	Pediatric surgery	48	0.5
Maternal, fetal medicine	45	0.5	Thoracic surgery	88	1.0
Reproductive endocrinology	64	0.7	Urology	117	1.3
Ophthalmology	332	3.8	No response	53	0.6
Orthopedic surgery	529	6.0	Total	8,809	100.0%

Source: Association of American Medical Colleges.

1980 (Table 4.10). Corrected for inflation, average indebtedness has increased by a factor of .7.

Medical school tuitions have risen steadily (Table 4.11), and the increased dependence on tuition revenues by private schools and many public schools is likely to force educational debts upward at an accelerated rate. The debt

Table 4.10   Mean Debt of Indebted Senior Medical Students, 1970-1981

| Academic year | Seniors with debt | | Percentage of seniors with debt |
	Current dollars	1979 dollars	
1970-1971	$ 5,500	$10,295	72%
1974-1975	9,000	13,265	71
1977-1978	13,800	16,552	76
1978-1979	15,800	17,612	76
1979-1980	17,212	17,212	77
1980-1981	19,697	17,670	77

Source: Association of American Medical Colleges.

Table 4.11   Summary of Average Tuitions of Selected Schools, 1960-1980

	1960	1980	Growth factor
Most expensive public	$ 776	$ 4,885	6.3
Least expensive public	267	573	2.1
Most expensive private	1,298	12,565	9.7
Least expensive private	868	5,830	6.7
Ratio			
High public, low public	2.9	8.5	
High private, low private	1.5	2.2	
High private, high public	1.7	2.6	
Low private, low public	3.3	10.2	

Source: Association of American Medical Colleges.

burden may be further enlarged because students have to turn to lending programs that carry a high rate of interest and little or no interest subsidy while they are in school.

The expansion of the faculties is slowing, and concerns are mounting about the reduction in openings for young faculty. Well-trained young clinical investigators are in particularly short supply. The increasing competition for research grants, coupled with pressures on clinical faculty to earn and share income from practice, makes opportunities in private practice more attractive than academic posts to young physicians whose counterparts in the 1960s and early 1970s sought careers in academic medicine. Under present tenure and retirement policies, slowing of growth means that there will be a progressive aging of the faculty. In 1980, 42 percent of the faculty were under forty years of age, and 25 percent were over fifty. By 1990, with zero growth, these proportions will be reversed.

The expansion of faculties, which exceeded the increase in students, has resulted in dispersion of responsibility for the undergraduate medical education program. In both the preclinical and clinical phases, multiple faculty members participate in courses and clerkships. As a result, even though the faculty/medical student ratio has increased, both the faculties and students complain of a lack of personal relationship between them. Students are also distressed because many courses consist of a parade of specialists and subspecialists, each lecturing on his own area in depth, with little overall coordination by a responsible course leader. The participation of an increased number of specialized faculty in the instruction of medical students is directly related to the explosion of biomedical knowledge with direct relevance to medical care that has occurred simultaneously with the expansion of the country's medical education capacity. Faced with the need to teach complex subjects to larger and larger classes, faculties have used available time for lectures and reduced or eliminated laboratory experience. There is a growing awareness that efforts must be made to identify essential knowledge and reduce the information load that students are expected to assimilate. In a recent survey, 56 percent of 515 faculty members answered *yes* to the question "Is the amount of information taught during the preclinical phase excessive, requiring too many lectures and conferences?" Another result of the dispersion of responsibility is a feeling that medical school faculties are not emphasizing sufficiently the importance of caring attitudes and respect for human needs. This was the perception of 71 percent of the faculty members surveyed.

The Future

The widely publicized forecast of an excess supply of physicians in the 1990s has not as yet had a major impact on the articulated program plans of institutions or on the career plans of students now in college. A recent straw poll of deans indicated that only about twelve schools are presently considering reductions in the size of their entering class.

APPLICANTS AND MATRICULANTS

During the 1970s the ratio of the number of medical and dental school applicants each year to the number of college freshmen who had indicated a probable career in medicine or dentistry four years earlier varied from a high of .73 in 1973 to a low of .41 in 1978. Since 1976 the ratio has fluctuated between .41 and .50. Projections through 1985, based on the indicated plans of students now in college, are shown in Table 4.12. It should be noted that the freshmen entering college in the fall of 1981 were the first class exposed to the projections of the Graduate Medical Education National Advisory Committee (GMENAC) report. Fewer of these students indicated an interest in medicine as a probable career choice. This is reflected in a drop in the number of applicants projected for 1985, which may be related to the high level of media discussion of a potential physician excess.

Table 4.12   *Projections of Medical School Applicants Based on Ratio of the Number of Freshmen Indicating Plans for a Career in Medicine to the Number of Applicants Four Years Later*

Ratio	1981	1982	1983	1984	1985
.5		37,830	36,830	37,650	35,550
	36,720 (actual)				
.4		30,260	29,460	30,125	28,440

Source: Association of American Medical Colleges.

The number of applicants to medical school has tended to parallel the number of 22-year-olds in the population. Exceptions to this trend occurred after World War II with the return of older veterans, and in the mid-1970s when the number of applicants reached an all-time high. In the mid-1980s a downturn in the size of the 22-year-old cohort will begin and will continue to the end of the century. This reduction in youth of college graduating age will doubtlessly be accompanied by a decreased number of medical school applicants. Superimposed on this demographic certainty are the effects of the increasing cost of medical education and changes in college students' perceptions of the desirability of a medical career with the forecast of a physician excess. Both are expected to depress the number of applicants.

Although the average age of medical school applicants has been shifting upward during the past decade, it is not likely that a downturn in the number of college students applying to medical school upon graduation will be offset by further growth in older applicants. In 1972, 66 percent of the applicants were 23 years of age or younger. By 1977 the proportion was 62 percent, and it dropped to 55 percent in 1980. The age range with the greatest increase was 24–27, which comprised 23 percent of applicants in 1972 and 30 percent in 1980. The major reason for this age shift is the fact that women tend to make somewhat later decisions to apply to medical school. There has been only a 1 percent increase in applicants 32 years of age or older. It does not appear likely that the decrease in 22-year-old applicants will be compensated by an increase in older applicants who make very late decisions to pursue a medical career. The increasing cost of attending medical school, coupled with perceptions that a financially secure career as a physician may not be assured due to possible physician oversupply, may be an even greater deterrent to older than to younger applicants.

There is no prior experience upon which to base forecasts of the influence of the increasing physician supply on women and minority applicants and matriculants. The number of women (both white and minority) has grown rapidly. Between 1970 and 1980 women matriculants increased 287 percent, while men increased only 19 percent. Thus far, the rate of increase in women applicants has not slowed. Whether women will view the anticipated physician excess as a deterrent to entering medicine to the same degree as men is conjectural. It is noteworthy that 20 percent of the 1981 women graduates, but only 10 percent of the men, indicated that their first career choice was a salaried clinical position in a hospital, group clinic, or government agency, and that 26 percent of the women, as opposed to 21 percent of the men, designated an academic career as their first choice. If the enlarged physician supply is coupled with a decrease in private practice opportunities and an expansion of salaried positions, women may become an even larger proportion of applicants and matriculants.

As noted earlier, the minority applicant pool rose quickly in the early 1970s and plateaued. One reason for lack of continued increases in the number of minority applicants is the high monetary and time costs of a medical education. There are many opportunities for capable minority students to enter other fields that require shorter and less-costly periods of education. The expanding physician supply, together with a decrease in financial support, will probably lower the number of qualified minority applicants. Financial resources to assist minority students are particularly important if this adverse trend is to be countered. Eighty percent of the 1981 minority graduates indicated that they had received scholarship support, compared with 45 percent of other graduates. Minority graduates had mean debt levels 5 percent greater than non-minorities.

As the applicant pool shrinks and the number of applicants per position diminishes, the academic quality of matriculants is likely to decline. Historically, the ratio of applicants to matriculants has approximated 2. When in 1960 the ratio fell to 1.7, the faculties of many schools expressed concern about the quality of some of the students they had to accept to fill their entering classes. The low applicant projection for 1985 shown in Table 4.11 will result in a ratio of 1.7, if the entering class size stays at the 1981 level.

There is considerable competition for desirable candidates among the medical schools. Only 17,286 of the 36,727 applicants for the 1981 entering class received an acceptance from a school. Of these, 626 did not matriculate in any school. It is apparent that the schools are competing for a restricted number of candidates who are perceived to be desirable by admissions committees. Schools' success in matriculating candidates to whom they offer positions is quite variable, ranging from 94 percent to 30 percent. The mean for public schools is 76 percent and for private schools, 50 percent (Table 4.13).

The public schools with the highest percentage of matriculants among their acceptees are those which are the only school in the state. In states where several public schools compete for a restricted applicant pool of state residents, each school has a lower percentage of acceptees who matriculate. Of particular interest are states with a long-established school and where a new school has recently been opened. The new school usually has significantly less success in attracting matriculants.

The overall lesser success of private schools in attracting matriculants is presumably due to their high tuitions. Within this group, however, the highest tuition schools are not necessarily the least successful.

As the applicant pool decreases and the cost of medical education rises, the competition for acceptable candidates can be expected to intensify. Single, long-established state schools will probably continue to have reasonable success in attracting satisfactory matriculants from their state residential pool of applicants because of their reputations and lower tuition. In states with multiple schools it is likely that more recently established schools will be less competitive. Overall, the private schools will fare less well than the public.

The competitive position of private schools may be further impaired by the withdrawal of state subsidies. During the era of expansion, many private schools were granted state subsidies to encourage their enrollment of in-state residents. Table 4.14 shows the state funds provided in support of both public and private medical schools in 1979. In sixteen states, private schools received state support ranging from a high of $23 million in Pennsylvania, to a low of $90 thousand in New Hampshire. This support is likely to be reduced or withdrawn as the expanding physician supply damps the concern about the need for additional physicians within states. The need to maintain support for the public schools within most states, combined with increasing

Table 4.13   Average Percentage of Acceptees that Matriculated,
             Based on Entering Classes of 1981, 1980, 1979

	Frequency	
Range	Public medical schools	Private medical schools
95-100	–	–
90-94	5	–
85-89	6	1
80-84	9	–
75-79	3	3
70-74	11	1
65-69	7	2
60-64	10	3
55-59	4	3
50-54	3	11
45-49	5	9
40-44	5	7
35-39	5	8
30-34	1	3
25-29	–	–
Total number of schools	74	51
Median	67.0%	49.0%
Mean	76.4%	50.1%
Range	94% - 30%	87% - 30%

Source: Association of American Medical Colleges.

demands on limited state resources for other obligations, will hasten withdrawal of state support from private schools. As a result, private school tuitions will be driven upward at a faster rate, making them progessively less competitive.

Multi-school states will face particularly hard decisions as the expanded physician supply decreases the pressure for maintenance of current enrollments in state institutions. As these states' resources for the support of their medical schools become more constrained, the decision to close one or more schools versus the decision to contract the enrollment in all schools and diminish the resources available for their programs equally will cause contentious debate. Maintaining program quality in fewer schools, a desirable outcome, may not be the political decision made in all states. This may lead to contention between state agencies and the Liaison Committee on Medical

Table 4.14   State Funds in Support of the State's Public and Private Medical Schools, 1979
(in thousands of dollars)

State	Public	Private
Total	$1,000,613	$79,446
Alabama	42,913	
Arizona	14,339	
Arkansas	8,507	
California	102,704	
Colorado	8,205	
Connecticut	11,613	
Florida	26,047	5,825
Georgia	17,426	1,837
Hawaii	7,087	
Illinois	48,406	6,742
Indiana	21,872	
Iowa	12,919	
Kansas	29,183	
Kentucky	16,918	
Louisiana	24,682	619
Maryland	14,518	356
Massachusetts	12,242	286
Michigan	48,490	
Minnesota	19,899	1,160
Mississippi	13,339	
Missouri	13,919	
Nebraska	14,008	
Nevada	1,474	90
New Hampshire		
New Jersey	32,056	
New Mexico	8,570	
New York	64,411	13,794
North Carolina	30,132	2,274
North Dakota	6,071	
Ohio	43,994	4,841
Oklahoma	13,000	
Oregon	10,039	
Pennsylvania	3,389	23,012
Puerto Rico	8,817	
Rhode Island		1,000
South Carolina	25,200	
South Dakota	2,879	
Tennessee	23,265	
Texas	128,290	12,693
Utah	5,496	
Vermont	3,910	
Virginia	31,407	1,208
Washington	n.a.	n.a.
West Virginia	17,684	
Wisconsin	11,293	3,709

Source: Association of American Medical Colleges.

Education because of failure of schools to maintain programs of sufficient quality to meet accreditation standards.

COMPETITION IN MEDICAL SERVICES

As state support of the medical schools diminishes, public institutions and many private schools will become increasingly dependent upon revenues generated by their faculties from the provision of medical services. This will create mounting competition between academic medical centers and community physicians and hospitals for patient care revenue. The expanded physician supply in the environs of the centers will intensify the competition for patients.

Historically, the academic centers have been able to provide medical services perceived to be of higher quality and complex specialized services not available elsewhere. Through their graduate medical education programs, the academic centers are now turning out well-educated and well-trained specialists and subspecialists who, upon completion, enter practice and compete with their former mentors. As the density of these competitors increases in the local environment, and as all types of specialists are distributed more widely across the landscape, referrals to many academic centers may decrease and their revenues from medical services may become limited. Some centers, because of their large research programs, will continue to attract patients because they will offer new services that are available nowhere else.

It is conceivable that lack of opportunity to open a private practice may make it attractive for well-trained, young physicians to seek appointments in the academic centers. While this could reverse the trend toward the loss of talented clinical investigators to private practice, the schools may not have the space or other resources to accommodate them. Older, tenured, but less productive faculty will not be inclined to leave their secure positions in academic centers to enter the competitive race in the community. Overall, 50 percent of the members of full-time faculties are tenured; in many institutions the proportion is significantly higher.

FACULTY AND PROGRAM

The fourfold expansion in faculty compared to a twofold increase in medical students during the past twenty years suggests that a decrease in enrollment may not be correlated with a parallel decrease in faculty. For the maintenance of basic science faculties, the future support of biomedical research will be the critical issue, and the needed income from medical services provided by clinical faculty will inhibit reductions in the size of clinical departments. The heavy engagement of clinical departments with graduate medical education will also deter reductions in clinical faculties as the undergraduate student body shrinks.

A decrease in the number of full-time medical school faculty would not necessarily harm the quality of undergraduate medical education. The dispersion of responsibility for medical education among a large number of faculty has tended to be depersonalizing. Consolidation of responsibility among a smaller faculty could actually improve educational quality if the staff is composed of effective, dedicated teachers.

Conclusion

Public perception of the pending increase in the supply of physicians will likely lead to a reduction in applicants and matriculants that could be rather precipitous by the mid-1980s. The proportion of female applicants and matriculants is expected to increase. The proportion of minorities may decrease, particularly if financial assistance is diminished.

Changes in the size of medical school faculties will not parallel the reduction in the medical student body. If biomedical research support is maintained, basic science faculties will continue to be sizable. The dependence upon revenue from the provision of medical services by clinical faculty will tend to maintain large clinical departments. States with several public schools and states that provide subsidies to private schools will have to make difficult political decisions about how to reduce and consolidate their support for the medical schools within their jurisdictions.

The anticipated reduction in class size could improve the quality of medical education if a limited number of capable faculty members assume responsibility for the academic medical centers' undergraduate medical education programs.

Appendix 4A Medical Schools Organized in the United States
            Since 1940

School	Year organized	1981 entering class
	1940-1949	
University of Texas, Southwestern Medical School, Dallas Texas	1943	205
University of Washington School of Medicine Seattle, Washington	1945	175
University of Puerto Rico, School of Medicine, San Juan	1949	150
	1950-1959	
University of California, Los Angeles, School of Medicine Los Angeles, California	1951	160
University of Miami, School of Medicine, Miami, Florida	1952	135
University of Kentucky, College of Medicine, Lexington, Kentucky	1954	108
Albert Einstein College of Medicine of Yeshiva University, New York, New York	1955	178
University of Florida, College of Medicine, Gainesville, Florida	1956	113
University of Medicine and Dentistry of New Jersey, New Jersey Medical School, Newark, New Jersey	1956	170
	1960-1969	
University of New Mexico, School of Medicine, Albuquerque, New Mexico	1960	73
University of California, Irvine College of Medicine Irvine, California	1962	98
University of Massachusetts, Medical School, Worcester, Massachusetts	1962	102
State University of New York, Stony Brook, School of Medicine Stony Brook, New York	1962	76
Brown University, Program in Medicine, Providence, Rhode Island	1963	61
Medical College of Ohio at Toledo Toledo, Ohio	1964	148
University of South Florida, College of Medicine, Tampa, Florida	1965	95
Louisiana State University, School of Medicine in Shreveport Shreveport, Louisiana	1966	103

School	Year organized	1981 entering class
	1960-1969	
Michigan State University College of Human Medicine East Lansing, Michigan	1966	104
University of Medicine and Dentistry of New Jersey, Rutgers Medical School, Piscataway, New Jersey	1966	130
University of South Alabama, College of Medicine, Mobile, Alabama	1967	64
University of Arizona, College of Medicine, Tucson, Arizona	1967	88
University of Hawaii John A. Burns School of Medicine Honolulu, Hawaii	1967	67
University of Nevada, School of Medical Sciences, Reno, Nevada	1967	48
Pennsylvania State University College of Medicine Hershey, Pennsylvania	1967	98
University of California, Davis School of Medicine Davis, California	1968	100
University of California, San Diego School of Medicine La Jolla, California	1968	125
University of Connecticut, School of Medicine, Farmington, Connecticut	1968	80
University of Missouri, Kansas City School of Medicine Kansas City, Missouri	1968	97
Mount Sinai School of Medicine of the City University of New York New York, New York	1968	100
University of Texas Medical School at San Antonio San Antonio, Texas	1968	202
Southern Illinois University School of Medicine Springfield, Illinois	1969	72
University of Texas, Medical School at Houston, Houston Texas	1969	202
Texas Tech University, School of Medicine, Lubbock, Texas	1969	100

(continued on next page)

Appendix 4A (continued)

School	Year organized	1981 entering class
	1970–1979	
Rush Medical College of Rush University, Chicago, Illinois	1971	119
Mayo Medical School Rochester, Minnesota	1971	40
University of Minnesota, School of Medicine, Duluth, Minnesota	1972	48
Eastern Virginia Medical School Norfolk, Virginia	1973	96
Uniformed Services University of the Health Sciences, School of Medicine, Bethesda, Maryland	1976	154
Wright State University, School of Medicine, Dayton, Ohio	1976	100
Universidad Central del Caribe* Escuela de Medicina Cayey, Puerto Rico	1976	68
East Carolina University, School of Medicine, Greenville, North Carolina	1977	52
Northeastern Ohio Universities, College of Medicine, Rootstown, Ohio	1977	92
University of South Carolina, School of Medicine, Columbia, South Carolina	1977	51
Texas A & M University, College of Medicine, College Station, Texas	1977	32
Ponce School of Medicine Ponce, Puerto Rico	1978	60
Marshall University School of Medicine Huntington, West Virginia	1978	36
Morehouse School of Medicine* Atlanta, Georgia	1978	32
Oral Roberts University* School of Medicine Tulsa, Oklahoma	1978	48
East Tennessee State University* College of Medicine Johnson City, Tennessee	1978	49

*Provisional accreditation

Source: Association of American Medical Colleges.

5

Medical Residencies in a Period of Expanding Physician Supply

DALE L. HIESTAND

This chapter will focus on the struggles and conflicts that may be precipitated within the residency system as a consequence of the ongoing rapid increase in the supply of physicians. Before examining that issue, however, several recent changes that have affected residency training should be noted.

First, the number of physicians graduating from medical schools and seeking to enter residency training programs has expanded rapidly since the late 1960s, and promises to continue to increase, though at a lesser rate. In 1983 there were 124 fully accredited medical schools in the United States, two with provisional accreditation, and one accredited to offer the first two years of the medical curriculum.[1] While there may be uncertainty about the exact effect that the schools still in the process of evolution will have on the supply of new physicians, the actual number of graduates from American medical schools may not increase very rapidly after the mid-1980s and could even decline. Nevertheless, the expectation is for nearly 17,000 applicants from this source for first-year residencies for the indefinite future.

As the expansion of American medical schools slowed in the late 1970s, increasing numbers of students sought a medical education abroad. Some returned via the Fifth Pathway program to complete their undergraduate training in American schools before residency. A growing number have applied for residencies without any preliminary training in an American school. As Table 5.1 indicates, the number of American citizens graduated from schools abroad (USFMGs) who apply for residencies is approximately 2,000 per year, compared to only 500 or less as recently as 1980. It may well reach 2,500 in the years ahead.

To these must be added the increasing pool of graduates of schools of osteopathy, a larger number of whom are seeking to enter both osteopathic and medical residencies than in previous years. Since 1978, five new schools of osteopathy have begun to graduate students, and all nine of the older schools also enlarged the size of their graduating classes. The number of

Table 5.1 Number of Applicants and First-Year Positions
          Reported by the National Residency Matching Program
          1952-1982

Year	Graduates of U.S. medical schools	USFMGs, (includes Fifth Pathway)	Total graduates of U.S. medical schools, USFMGs	First-year positions offered	Positions per total U.S. grads, USFMGs
1952	6,089	---	6,089	10,414	1.71
1953	6,668	---	6,668	10,971	1.65
1954	6,861	---	6,861	10,729	1.56
1955	6,977	---	6,977	11,075	1.59
1956	6,845	---	6,845	11,459	1.67
1957	6,796	---	6,796	11,804	1.74
1958	6,861	---	6,861	11,958	1.74
1959	6,860	---	6,860	12,250	1.79
1960	7,081	---	7,081	12,390	1.75
1961	6,994	---	6,994	12,686	1.81
1962	7,168	---	7,168	12,705	1.77
1963	7,264	---	7,264	12,456	1.71
1964	7,336	---	7,336	12,601	1.72
1965	7,409	---	7,409	13,038	1.76
1966	7,574	---	7,574	13,463	1.78
1967	7,743	---	7,743	14,178	1.83
1968	7,973	---	7,973	14,566	1.83
1969	8,059	---	8,059	15,045	1.87
1970	8,367	---	8,367	15,567	1.86
1971	8,974	---	8,974	16,515	1.84
1972	9,551	---	9,551	17,283	1.81
1973	10,391	---	10,391	18,721	1.80
1974	11,613	89	11,702	17,403	1.49
1975	12,714	151	12,865	15,691	1.22
1976	13,561	297	13,858	16,112	1.16
1977	13,607	340	13,947	16,574	1.19
1978	14,393	403	14,796	17,219	1.16
1979	14,966	458	15,424	17,824	1.16
1980	15,135	506	15,641	18,055	1.15
1981	15,667	1,241	16,908	18,331	1.08
1982	16,281	1,876	18,157	18,300	1.01

Source: National Residency Matching Program, Evanston, Ill.

osteopathic graduates, which came to 1,004 in 1978–1979, is expected to exceed 1,800 by 1989–1990.[2]

The initial rapid expansion in the numbers applying for residencies was outpaced by an even more rapid expansion in the number of residency positions. The discrepancy was at its height in the late 1960s and early 1970s, and the gap was largely filled by noncitizen graduates of foreign medical schools (FMGs). More recently, the number of noncitizen graduates of foreign medical schools applying for residencies declined from nearly 6,000 in 1976 to 2,000 or less in 1979, 1980, and 1981. In 1982, however, their number jumped to 3,500.[3] This is thought to reflect the discovery of paths to circumvent the restrictive legislation of 1976, including the provision of entry preference for the spouse of an alien legally residing in the United States.

As Table 5.1 indicates, the number of first-year residency positions offered currently is now in excess of the total of applicants from American schools and U.S. citizens graduated from foreign schools. This does not include graduates of osteopathic schools nor the new wave of FMGs attempting to enter medical residencies. Most osteopathic graduates enter osteopathic internships, which have been increasing, but a rising number of osteopathic graduates are being accepted in allopathic residencies.[4]

Thus we are now passing through a period in which the supply/demand equation for first-year residents is shifting into a position of excess supply. Indeed, the number of first-year residencies offered seems to fluctuate unpredictably.[5] Given the expected continued increase in the number of applicants, we are at some kind of a watershed, with consequences that cannot be anticipated fully.

Whether medical school graduates are spending more or less time in graduate medical education is not clear. Surely there has been an increase over the long run, as specialists have substantially replaced general practitioners. In recent years, the trends have been mixed. The internship has been abolished. Preparation for some specialties has been lengthened; for others, shortened. The proportion selecting surgical and other nonprimary care programs has remained almost constant, about 60 percent, despite considerable effort to encourage the training of primary care physicians.[6] Many who start out to become primary physicians later decide to pursue more advanced specialty training. There has been anecdotal evidence in the last year or so that some subspecialty programs are losing support and are shrinking or being allowed to expire. Thus it is uncertain whether the average number of years in graduate medical education is increasing or decreasing.

The total number of physicians undertaking graduate medical education, which expanded rapidly throughout the 1960s and 1970s, declined 5 percent from 1979 to 1980, then rose a precipitous 11 percent in 1981, and currently seems to be continuing to increase, though at a slower rate.[7] As Table 5.2 shows, between 1979 and 1982 there was significant growth in the number of

Table 5.2   Number of Residents on Duty September 1, 1979, 1980, 1981, and 1982 by Specialty

Specialty	Residents on Duty			
	1979	1980	1981	1982
Allergy, immunology	155	192	203	236
Anesthesiology	2,491	2,490	2,930	3,369
Colon, rectal surgery	42	37	40	46
Dermatology	801	755	814	789
Dermatopathology	19	30	30	35
Emergency medicine[b]	--	--	--	885
Family practice	6,352	6,344	7,004	7,040
Internal medicine	16,580	15,964	17,537	17,185
Neurological surgery	579	511	608	621
Neurology	1,212	1,114	1,236	1,276
Nuclear medicine	174	176	197	203
Obstetrics-gynecology	4,496	4,221	4,705	4,702
Ophthalmology	1,538	1,480	1,543	1,553
Orthopedic surgery	2,572	2,418	2,667	2,733
Otolaryngology	1,038	923	995	1,001
Pathology	2,519	2,186	2,413	2,437
Blood banking	21	23	26	32
Forensic	24	22	31	28
Neuropathology	52	52	41	37
Pediatrics	5,603	5,171	5,961	5,720
Allergy	53	2[a]	--	--
Cardiology	128	130	111	104
Physical medicine, rehabilitation	490	492	605	624
Plastic surgery	412	367	389	365
Preventive medicine				
General	199	157	166	188
Aerospace medicine	25	25	43	46
Occupational medicine	70	71	75	78
Public health	23	31	25	31
Psychiatry	3,901	3,911	4,336	4,235
Child	521	426	501	528
Radiology diagnostic	3,024	2,766	3,135	3,155
Diagnostic (nuclear)	45	48	58	62
Therapeutic	377	288	352	388
Surgery	7,689	7,440	8,105	8,064
Pediatric	37	29	27	27
Thoracic surgery	276	256	281	278
Urology	1,077	917	1,027	1,041
Total	64,615	61,465	68,217	69,142

[a]Many pediatric allergy programs were reaccredited as allergy and immunology.
[b]Emergency medicine was added to the specialty count in 1982.
Source: Journal of the American Medical Association. 1983.
         250(12):1545.

residents in anesthesiology; family practice and internal medicine also made substantial gains. The largest absolute losses in the number of residents occurred in pathology, plastic surgery, otolaryngology, and urology.

The number and proportion of residents who are women has increased rapidly, reflecting the growth in the number of women entering and graduating from American medical schools, as well as the decline in the number of noncitizens, a greater proportion of whom have been male. By 1982, more than 23 percent of all residents were women.[8] The number of residents who are members of minority groups has increased slightly. These changes have paralleled the earlier increases in the representation of blacks and Hispanics in medical schools, and the recent plateauing at less than 5 percent for each group.[9] The characterization of Asians in this context is problematic for two reasons. First, few Asian-Americans can be considered disadvantaged minorities in the traditional sense. And second, Asian aliens constitute a major fraction of noncitizen FMGs participating in American residency programs.[10]

Implications

The preceding analysis points to the rapidly changing supply/demand conditions with respect to medical residencies. Clearly, to the extent that the balance shifts, rates of change and timing will differ by field of practice and specialization, geographic location, mode of practice, and institutional setting. One can anticipate a variety of scenarios in different settings that will alter the parameters of the system as a whole and the way in which various parts of it respond. A variety of conflict points among different groups of physicians and different parts of the institutional structure are likely to emerge, with direct effects on the residency system and its components.

These conflict situations and their attendant scenarios can be conceptualized as arising via the market system, via governmental actions, or via organizational actions. In the real world, of course, actions in each of these three arenas are intermingled over time and are mutually interactive.

The most elementary proposition from market theory is that continued increases in the supply of physicians, relative to the population and the demand for services, will tend to lower (or at least decelerate) average real incomes of physicians. This is true even though individual physicians and groups of physicians may be able to influence the demand for their services. The reduction or slow growth of real income per physician can generally be expected to lower the incentives to enter medicine and undergo a long period of postgraduate training. In this sense, the market is a self-adjusting, self-correcting mechanism that would bring the number seeking residencies into balance with the opportunities to enter residencies and practice.

Alternatively, the newer graduates because of greater skill, enterprise, etc., could gain a share in the medical marketplace large enough to maintain incentives to enter and complete medical school and graduate medical education. In this scenario, the losses in income would be concentrated among older physicians, who would tend to experience declining practices and early retirement.

It is entirely consistent with market theory that difficulties confronting the young in gaining entry and satisfactory incomes in the medical marketplace would be an incentive for them to extend the length of time they spend in training in order to intensify their skills and area of specialization. The resultant highly trained specialists would thus become more attractive to patients and potential colleagues for referrals, partnerships, and other group arrangements.

There is anecdotal evidence that younger physicians are encountering increasing difficulty in finding a suitable practice opportunity and building a practice. There is also anecdotal evidence that older physicians are confronted by increasing competition for patients. Yet, there is no conclusive evidence to date that physicians in general are suffering reduced real incomes and reduced incentives as a result of competition from greater numbers. Real income per physician did decline irregularly after 1974, as Table 5.3 indicates. Dollar incomes increased, but not as fast as the overall inflation rate. Whether the failure of physicians' incomes to keep pace with inflation in the late 1970s reflected a decline in the relative attractiveness of the profession may be questioned.

Table 5.3   *Physicians' Average Income, 1974–1979*

	Current dollars	1974 dollars
1974	$54,140	$54,140
1975	58,440	53,600
1976	62,800	54,400
1977	65,430	53,200
1978	68,040	51,400
1979	76,720	52,400

Source: *Medical Economics,* September 17, 1979; September 15, 1980; September 28, 1981 (adapted).

The incomes of those in other fields also lagged the inflation that OPEC-induced energy costs spread throughout the economy. Also, the rapid increase in the number of physicians shifted the age distribution of the total supply so that larger numbers and a larger proportion were in the early years of establishing a practice, when incomes could be expected to be low. The real test will be their success in building a practice to provide a high income over the longer run. Finally, more and more entrants into practice have located in regions and smaller cities where the cost of living tends to be lower; this factor raises questions about the validity of comparisons between their incomes and national price indices.

Real income did lag in particular fields, such as general surgery, obstetrics-gynecology, and pediatrics, pointing perhaps to temporary surpluses in those fields, given present spending patterns. Although the incentives to enter those specialties may have been reduced, paradoxically, the number of first-year residents has shown a slight rise.

Of course, it is *expected* income that constitutes the financial motive to opt for a medical career. Those who are partway through their medical education have strong incentives to complete it, even though their expectations may be declining. Although prevailing incomes are often the best clue available to young people concerning ultimate rewards in a field, the possibility or probability of future "surpluses" of physicians is gaining currency as successive reports, forecasts, and analyses are published. Moreover, any declining incentives would manifest themselves first in lagging interest in premedical programs and medical schools. Adjustments via the marketplace that serve to reduce interest in a medical career would be apparent long before they affected residency programs.

Only if income and related incentives actually collapsed would there be any significant stimulus for medical school graduates or those in the residency stream to seek other fields of employment. That may yet occur, but no current evidence points in this direction. Indeed, the surge in the late 1970s of Americans studying at foreign medical schools and their efforts to enter residencies and practice in the U.S. is testimony to continued high incentives. This is particularly true in view of current poor opportunities for persons of high potential to enter fields that conceivably compete with medicine, with the possible exception of business, law, and computers.

A variety of "nonmarket" or policy responses might affect the residency system as a result of rapidly increasing numbers of physicians and the growing perception of a possible "oversupply." Among these are policies affecting the allocation of monies for residency training, the policies of established specialists and their professional associations with respect to the accreditation and maintenance of residency programs, the staffing policies of hospitals with respect to the services presently performed by residents, and public and private policies governing the entry of foreign-trained physicians into American residencies.

The costs of residency training have been considered a legitimate component of the rate base or allowable expenses of teaching hospitals for claims submitted to Blue Cross and other insurance systems, Medicare, and Medicaid. At the same time, there has been considerable public and organizational debate about the rising costs of health services in general, conceptualized as the need for "cost containment." The issue is whether, in light of the increasing supply of physicians, initiatives to review more closely or disallow certain residency costs may be undertaken by the various public and private bodies that set the rates and absorb the costs of hospital care. This might include federal executive or legislative initiatives with respect to Medicare and Medicaid; similar state initiatives with respect to Medicaid, Blue Cross, and other hospital insurance rates; and initiatives by Blue Cross, other private insurers, and the hospitals themselves. New York State authorities sought to review the appropriateness of charges for residency programs included in Medicaid reimbursements in 1980, but the effort was successfully challenged on the basis of the legality of the particular review mechanism. Maryland recently began to justify the establishment of certain special surgery units in nonteaching hospitals on the grounds of lower costs, which tend to undercut the financial support for related residency programs in teaching hospitals. Other steps may be taken by the federal or state governments or private organizations to limit or even reduce the financial support for residencies that will lead to selective erosion of the scale of the system.

The pressure for cost containment may also come via the marketplace. Health insurance accounts for a large part of the cost of employee fringe benefits. Both employers and unions are showing increased interest in cost containment in the health industry. For instance, the issue has recently been on the agenda of the Business Roundtable. This concern promises to be one more threat to the finances of teaching hospitals and thus to graduate medical education.

This is related, in turn, to emerging problems in maintaining adequate flows of patients in teaching hospitals to support residency programs. As the number of specialists has increased throughout the nation, and as the newer supply has tended to locate in the suburbs, smaller cities, and outlying areas, patients with somewhat complicated conditions and needs are less likely than in the past to be referred to tertiary teaching hospitals. Moreover, there is considerable pressure for the growth of HMOs, which may further lower hospitalization rates. Even in large cities, physicians are beginning to set up more freestanding surgical and emergency centers, independent of hospitals.

As a result, some teaching hospitals are facing problems in maintaining adequate patient flows to meet the numerical standards for an approved teaching base in various specialties. Some teaching hospitals are trying to organize residency programs that would extend into outlying areas. Whether or not these efforts are successful, there may well be increasing numbers of specialized residency programs that are unable to maintain the patient flow needed to qualify as a training site. Conflicts may arise among various kinds of advanced residency or fellowship programs over which sets of residents will have access to the patients for training purposes.

The major teaching hospitals (325 in all) already receive more than \$21 billion, or 28 percent of all dollars spent on hospital services.[10] Concentrated heavily in central cities, they tend to face major capital needs to keep apace of new technology and to replace aging and obsolescent facilities. They are also under constant pressures to provide community and emergency room services. While this contributes to the needed flow of patients for their teaching needs, it is also a severe burden on their budgets. In the future, cost containment pressures and competition for operating and capital resources may infringe seriously on graduate medical education.

Whether a group of specialists may undertake collective action via their professional societies to limit directly or indirectly the number of residencies and thus inhibit future competition is a question that is always present. In fact, conflicts may occur within particular specialty groups between those members who are interested in a teaching career and those who are practitioners, with the academicians, professional leaders, and association officials adopting varying positions. For instance, the organized medical profession is at present committed to the principle that the approval of particular residency programs should be based on qualitative considerations alone. In many nonmedical professional and educational areas, however, it is not unknown for individual officials to vary the stringency with which they apply qualitative standards in accordance with their perceptions of the need for the particular kinds of professionals being trained. While leaders of the medical profession may not support it, the possibility exists that determinations by individual teaching hospitals, department chairmen, review committees, etc., may be influenced by restrictive tendencies if the perception grows that supplies in selective specialties and localities are adequate. Those responsible for educational programs will be under increasing pressure from practicing specialists with regard to educational decisions, financing, etc.

Legal realities may make it extremely difficult for medical organizations to undertake many types of efforts to control the growth of medical manpower. Despite the evidence, organized medicine still is widely perceived to be restricting the supply and acting contrary to the public interest. Freedom of competition is being extended to professional fields, a right that is supported by a series of court decisions bearing on professional advertising, entry into practice, etc. The threat of intervention by the Federal Trade Commission and judicial authorities is widely considered to be real, although there is apparent conflict among the administration, the regulatory agencies, and the courts with respect to "pro-competition" and diminishing or intensifying antitrust activity.

In this connection, the competition among specialty groups must be considered. Any particular group that tries to restrict the supply within its own specialty may discover that other groups are only too willing to turn their talents to a wide array of cases that may quite logically be treated by either specialty. This does not mean that gynecologists will compete for brain surgery with neurological surgeons. But many cases are on the borderline between specialties. Neurologists compete with neurosurgeons in the care of certain conditions; some patients might feasibly be treated by a gynecologist or a general surgeon; the dividing line between cardiologists and internists is not precise. Thus, action by any particular group of specialists to limit their numbers by limiting residencies is always restrained by the fear of losing "turf." Each group also fears that attempts to restrict numbers may inhibit the development and dissemination of new techniques in their field, which is an important function of active teaching programs.

Finally, the changing supply of physicians and of other types of health manpower may induce certain hospitals (or make it easier for them) to reduce their range of residency programs. Hospitals are finding it less difficult to attract physicians for full-time and part-time salaried posts. They may therefore decide that the service needs now met by residents can be covered more satisfactorily by salaried staff. Alternatively, if the increasing supply means that individual specialists have relatively more free time in their practice, they may be willing to perform some of the services for their hospitalized patients that are the responsibility of residents. The pressure for cost containment might lead not only to the use of staff physicians, but also to the deployment of other health manpower groups, such as physician's associates and assistants, nurse practitioners, midwives, etc., for selected tasks now performed by residents. Montefiore Hospital, for instance, pioneered in the utilization of surgical assistants for functions often performed by residents.

The growing sense of a threat of an oversupply of physicians is certain to provoke continued controversy over the rights of graduates of both foreign and American schools to enter residency training. The history of investigatory, regulatory, and judicial actions and responses may only be prelude to more tortured future developments. Without tracing this record in detail, it may suffice to note that the controversy has been joined at international, national, state, and local levels, and involves immigration law and regulation; the availability of educational grants and loans for study abroad; the eligibility of alien FMGs and USFMGs for licenses and residencies; testing and Fifth Pathway mechanisms; the roles of state educational authorities and the American professional associations in the evaluation of foreign medical schools; and so on.

State Variations

A few of the major factors altering the future of the residency system are national in scope. Some examples are the posture of the federal government with respect to immigration and cost containment, and the policies and practices of national medical and other organizations. Most of the important changes, however, will take place within state and local governments and organizations, and in other small-area contexts. This raises the distinct probability that different scenarios will unfold in different settings. Recent postures and developments within a few states are suggestive.

New York State has consistently held what might be termed an expansionary stance toward the supply of physicians. It has the highest physician/population ratio of any state. It has a total of twelve academic medical centers. Of the six centers in New York City, two were established during the last three decades, and there is considerable support for the development of another. There are two new medical centers in the New York City suburbs, one of them by migration out of the city, the other wholly new. Of the four upstate medical centers, two were reorganized as units of the State University of New York (SUNY). Most of these centers, new or old, have expanded substantially during the last two decades, either within a particular complex of facilities or by affiliation agreements involving the establishment and/or direction of residency programs in neighboring hospitals. State government has exercised a major influence by assuming financial and operating responsibility for four medical schools. In addition, private funds have been mobilized to set up a school of osteopathy, with high-level political support.

New York State produces an unusually high proportion of young people who desire and actually gain entry to medical practice by undertaking undergraduate medical training and residencies both in and out of the state. They are the major source of American citizens studying abroad and seeking reentry to American medical schools, residencies, and practice. At the same time, New York has been a magnet for foreigners who have come for decades for medical school training, residencies, and/or practice. Despite vigorous resistance by the medical and educational establishments, both in and out of the state, the New York Board of Regents took the initiative in 1981 of inviting foreign medical schools to submit information regarding their programs to facilitate the evaluation of their American graduates who seek to enter New York's medical system.

Although New York's medical centers face continuing financial pressures, particularly the older institutions with capital plants in need of renovation, New York authorities were innovators in seeking to limit the flow of Medicaid funds into residencies. As noted above, the effort was overruled in the courts.

This is not to say that there is no concern in the state with respect to the continued growth of the physician manpower supply. There is, however, strong public and political support for expansion by both consumer and medical interests, often along ethnic, religious, and racial lines.

Indiana presents a quite different picture of a carefully managed medical educational system, with an unequivocal policy of avoiding overexpansion.

Indiana, in fact, is at about the national average in such indices as the physican/population ratio, the proportion of young people entering medical school, etc. It has a single medical school, the second-largest in the country. Very few Indiana citizens seek medical education outside the state, and very few out-of-staters enroll in its medical education program. All residencies in the state are conducted by the University of Indiana Medical School or are affiliated with it. It is a centrally managed system, with strong political and organizational support. Its characterization as a "lean" system is enhanced by such practices as a meticulous scrutiny of the time allocated by residents to different tasks, and pressures on attending physicians to perform their own "scut" work that might be delegated to residents elsewhere.

California has consistently imported physician manpower. It has eight academic medical centers, three privately funded and five public. Most of its medical school expansion has been in the state university system, which accepts very few nonresidents. Two of the three private schools receive one-half or more of their students from out of state. Planning for the system is vested primarily in the state government. The executive and the legislative leaders jointly agreed in 1979 to halt any further expansion of medical school capacity, and to depend for the future on in-migration of physicians who have received undergraduate training in other states for its much larger system of residencies. The attractive San Francisco Bay area has for some years had what is widely considered an oversupply of physicians. There, salaried positions continue to be avidly sought. In southern California, particularly in Orange County and the San Diego area, inflows of physicians from other states also continue. Various forms of HMOs are popular and relatively widespread in different parts of the state. As a matter of organizational policy and to contain costs, these systems and their affiliated hospitals as well as the private hospital chains have played only a limited role in graduate medical education.

Although California has long attracted a significant inflow of both citizen and noncitizen FMGs, that fact has never seemed to be as controversial as it is in the East. This may be due to the relative shortage of physicians in rapidly expanding areas in the southern part of the state and elsewhere. It may also reflect the fact that a large proportion of the state's population consists of Mexicans, Mexican-Americans, and various Asian and Asian-American groups. California is also unusual in the popularity and relative political strength of non-physician health providers, including nurses, midwives, and others. The threat of competition from these groups is a recurrent cause for concern in California medical circles.

New Jersey developed its medical education system relatively recently. It long depended upon the major medical centers in New York and Philadelphia, to which New Jersey residents turned for their medical care. More recently, the suburban areas of both north and south Jersey have acquired physicians from these metropolitan medical centers who continue to refer tertiary patients to their parent institutions, although in declining numbers.

Medical education in the state is concentrated in two medical centers, which are part of the state university system. Planning and expansion of the system have been careful and slow. There continues to be pressure for a third medical center in the south, which elicits partial and reluctant response at best. Many New Jersey residents go to other states for medical school and/or residencies, and many enter practice in other states. There has also been a significant flow of New Jersey residents to foreign medical schools. Many return to New Jersey hospitals for clinical clerkships and residencies, and their quality and credentials have been a continuing subject of debate. In sum, one might characterize New Jersey's policies with respect to physician manpower issues as cautious, planned, and concerned with state budgetary implications. New Jersey has pressed, for instance, for a relatively high share of the costs of medical education to be met by tuition, on the grounds that a medical career is highly rewarding to the individual.

Conclusion

It is worth noting that the residency system, despite its high degree of coherence, nevertheless is composed of a great many discrete, small parts. In 1982, there were 325 major teaching hospitals, some 37 recognized specialties or subspecialties, and 4,573 accredited residency programs, accommodating 69,142 residents. This averages out to about fourteen programs per major teaching hospital and some thirteen residents per program. Since most programs are for two or three years, a typical program may admit only five or six residents per year. These are only averages, however, and particular programs may admit as few as one (or none) or as many as fifty.

The essential fact is that nearly all residency programs are quite small, dealing with a limited number of quite distinctive individuals. Therefore, it is all the more problematic just how the highly complex set of market, public, and organizational forces and processes outlined above will affect the system as a whole, its many parts, and the individuals within it.

Seen in this light, it is perhaps too early to attempt any judgment of what the net outcome of the multiple processes, pressures, and conflicts will be. Perhaps because of its highly complex nature, institutional arrangements in the profession of medicine move very slowly, although there are significant turning points. To realize this one has only to recall the time required to effectuate the program envisioned in the Flexner report. The endless debate attending the evolution of health insurance over the past fifty years has turned on controversies over whether the program should be public or private; national or regional; comprehensive or categorical; and universal or for defined groups, such as employees, the aged, the poor. One might also cite the gradual evolution of the forms of financial support for the medical educational system as a whole over the past thirty years. Nevertheless, a number of critical turning points are evident at present, whose consequences are unpredictable.

Notes

1. *Journal of the American Medical Association.* 1983. 250(12):1509.
2. *The D.O.* 1981. 21(April):9. In 1968, there were only five osteopathic schools; 427 physicians were graduated that year.
3. National Resident Matching Program, unpublished data.
4. *The D.O.* 1981. 50–51.
5. *Journal of the American Medical Association.* 1983. 1546.
6. Steinwachs, D., et al. 1982. Changing Patterns of Graduate Medical Education. *New England Journal of Medicine* 306(1):10–14.
7. See *Journal of the American Medical Association.* 1983 and Table 5.1 for conflicting figures in recent years.
8. *Journal of the American Medical Association.* 1983. 1546.
9. *Journal of the American Medical Association.* 1983. 1550.
10. American Hospital Association. 1980 Annual Survey. Unpublished data.

6

Defining and Certifying the Specialists

ROSEMARY A. STEVENS

Any analysis of specialization must begin with the obvious, if frustrating, observation that there is no single definition of a specialty, nor, indeed, can there be outside of uniform, organized health care systems with specific job descriptions. As the Graduate Medical Education National Advisory Committee (GMENAC) Report noted, defining an individual's specialty depends on whether one is measuring "specialty" in terms of individual preference, choice, or attainment.[1] We might redefine these alternatives as what physicians say they wish to do, what they actually do, and what they are trained or certified to do—recognizing that these are not necessarily the same. Apart from some broad generalizations, I shall avoid the question of what it is individual physicians do, in terms of the units of time devoted to particular specialty activities and how these units may change in the future. Instead I shall concentrate on two broader, perhaps more policy-relevant aspects of medical specialization: (a) the changing role of specialty certification, and (b) the definition of specialist fields as the marketplace becomes more challenging and more limiting. The latter would include the labeling and marketing of new fields.

Virtually every physician now in a residency expects to become certified in a specialty. There are now thirty-five residency training programs in the specialties, from aerospace medicine to urology, each leading to appropriate certification. While certification does not in itself imply a single choice of work or an array of specialist functions, board certification has been evolving into a system of specialist licensure. The number of residency positions available in each field clearly limits the supply of trained personnel in selected fields. For specialties such as ophthalmology, where the demand for residency training may exceed supply, the residency review process (i.e., the sum of decisions as to which residency programs are approved) acts as a powerful rationing device. Only an exceedingly rash physician would, for example, set up shop as an ophthalmologist without residency training in this field, if only for fear of charges of malpractice. Future directions in the combined residency review and certification process are thus central to thinking about trends in specialization.

But if certification is the formal process of specialty definition, self-label-ing and marketing of services or skills provide together a potent, informal source of specialization, designed directly to appeal to new consumers—whether these are patients, physicians, or other health practitioners. In an increasingly competitive marketplace successful specialists will be those who are seen to have most practical appeal.

Specialty labels have always been useful marketing devices, but specialists also have to create their markets—whether around machinery (the CT scanner, for example), techniques (emergency medicine), age groups (geria-trics), or conditions (obesity). A prospective patient with an arm sore from tennis might well choose a specialist in sports medicine over an internist or a general orthopedic surgeon, assuming the choice were available. But labeling is also important as a mark of prestige within medicine. A physician might disdain the label of geriatrician, on grounds of status, but develop a recog-nized niche as a consultant in nursing home care. An obstetrician-gynecologist might extend his/her range by setting up as a specialist in "climacteric problems"—and developing this field with flair. Questions of labeling and marketing are not the same as those traditionally considered under specialty preference, but I believe they will become more important in the future as the number of physicians increases.

Behind the two processes of specialist certification and specialty labeling is amore fundamental potential shift. I think that we shall see different notions of the *idea* of a specialty over the next few decades. As fields expand, divide, and recombine, certification by the traditional specialty boards will become less useful in defining and describing specialties. Most of the boards were, after all, developed before 1950. Specialist associations or certificates of spe-cial training, competence, or expertise—in wide fields such as nutrition or nursing home care, or narrow fields such as the hematology of leukemia—may give a future employer more information than whether a candidate is certified in internal medicine, psychiatry, pathology, or pediatrics. At the same time, the increasing tendency of physicians to accept salaried positions or to associate with partnerships will bring employment criteria to the fore. Large health maintenance organizations (HMOs) or health care chains may wish to designate or provide specified training in certain areas of practice, irrespective of the requirements of the boards. In any event, the definition of a specialty is likely to grow more dependent on sociocultural factors, includ-ing employment, and less on traditional professional processes. The role of board certification will come increasingly under question.

As a final general observation, it must be emphasized that specialization is heavily dependent on the organization and financing of health services. A city whose population is covered for the most part by HMOs can expect a system of specialists that is defined as the sum of decisions in the HMOs, with a "medical fringe" providing services not covered by the HMO, or acting as an additional form of private practice for patients who seek an outlet for one reason or another (e.g., convenience, to avoid long waiting time, privacy for a particular condition, doubt or distrust of HMO physicians, or a second opinion). This might be dubbed "Harley Street practice," in that it would play a somewhat similar role to private practice in the British National Health Service.

Alternatively, a large health insurance scheme (whether government-sponsored or industry-sponsored) might change the apparent balance of specialties in an area or population virtually overnight—by insisting, for example, that every beneficiary have a personal physician, or by allowing some specialist qualifications to draw in additional privileges or fees. Rather than attempt to allow for specific changes in the organization and financing of the health care system, or to create a unified picture of the "future," it makes more sense to consider the behavior of specialists and the processes of specialization as a series of possible scenarios or propositions.

The following propositions are presented as "best guesses" of what may happen to specialization if and as the number of physicians continues to increase. More general questions of specialist certification and specialty labeling will then be returned to.

1. *Increasing numbers of physicians will create demand within existing specialties to increase services within traditional fields.* We may expect to see, inter alia, an increased number of follow-up visits after an initial visit, a new focus on the annual physical examination and other preventive measures, an increased number of diagnostic tests and procedures, and a resistance to substitution of non-physician for physician services.

2. *The boundaries of traditional specialties will be extended.* We may expect to see, for example, general psychiatrists increasing their involvement in somatic illness; allergists extending their interest in psychosomatic medicine, rheumatologists moving into more general aches and pains, plastic surgeons confronting head and neck surgeons, urologists tackling more general questions of the male condition, endocrinologists converging upon clinical pharmacology, and so on. (These specialties are expected to run a "surplus" in 1990 under GMENAC projections.)

3. *Second opinions and referrals will increase.* Second opinion schemes for surgery can already be justified on grounds of quality of care, if not of cost. Demands for second opinions may be expected from physician groups, particularly as criticism of "excess surgery" continues. Medical and psychiatric opinions may also become more frequent as a natural corollary of proposed surgery. In office practice one-fourth of new patients are now referrals; this proportion may be expected to increase. The potential conflict between a referral system, whereby a physician may lose a patient to another physician, and an increasing tendency toward follow-up visits, whereby the physician

retains his/her own patients, will generate increased interest among physicians in given areas for mutual referral schemes and, more extensively, for well-defined referral networks. That is, a defined group of physicians will agree, formally or by custom, to refer among themselves, thus leading to self-defining service networks.

4. *As the number of services rises, there will be increased criticism of specialists on the grounds of rising costs and unnecessary services.* Specialist organizations will counter this criticism by conducting studies similar to the Study on Surgical Services for the United States (SOSSUS) and by at least lip service to outcome criteria. It must be remembered, however, that the SOSSUS findings have apparently had little effect on surgeon supply. (Surveys in Rhode Island, for example, show *more* surgeons in the state, more surgical procedures, and lighter operative work loads, despite SOSSUS.)[2] Thus, a period of intensive self-scrutiny by specialist groups may be followed by a period of renewed hostilities between purchasing groups and specialist associations.

5. *Some specialties will be able to accommodate an increasing supply of physicians by fostering narrower subspecialty fields.* In some cases we may see subspecialties of subspecialties. For example, in hematology, a subspecialty of internal medicine, we may expect a variety of modalities dealing with leukemia: hematology/oncology, hematology/coagulation, and hematology/white-cell diseases. Head and neck surgery, a subfield of surgery, is another example: head and neck oncology is already becoming a field of interest. Radiology has fostered nuclear medicine. We may also see an increased interest among diagnostic radiologists in noninvasive diagnostic and therapeutic techniques, and more recognition of the subfield of CT scan interpretation. Pathology has developed a whole series of subspecialty training programs in the last few years: in an atomic and clinical pathology, in neuropathology, in forensic pathology, in blood banking, in radioisotopic pathology and dermatopathology. These, too, may spawn esoteric subspecialties.

These concentrated fields, a recognition of a finer focus within existing fields, will lead an increasing number of physicians into superspecialties, based either on large multispecialist groups or, more probably, on academic medical centers.

Tertiary medical centers have a vested interest in proclaiming unique, specialized areas of competence. As medical schools are themselves subject to increased competition for scarce federal biomedical research funds, the rush to subspecialize will increase. Third-party payment schemes will find it difficult, if not impossible, to exclude such expertise from coverage.

6. *All else being equal, the proportion of primary care practitioners is likely to decrease.* The primary care market is difficult to predict. Approximately half of all residents in 1980–1981 were being trained in "primary care" fields of internal medicine, family practice, pediatrics, and obstetrics-gynecology. Yet there was also a decrease in the number of

residents in these fields, from more than 33,000 in 1979 to less than 32,000 in 1980. Moreover, many of the residents in these fields will not enter the practice of primary care and will choose, instead, a subspecialty field.

Assuming that the total number of first-year residency positions continues to decline (there was a decline from 18,702 Post Graduate-1 [PG1] positions in 1980–1981 to 17,602 in 1982–1983), fourth-year medical students will be constrained increasingly by the availability of positions in different specialty fields. There is no immediate sign of greater numerical or proportional preference for primary care via recognition in the specialist structure of residency training; quite the reverse. Changes in the policy of residency review, or in decisions about specialty mix in the medical schools, could obviously change this position. Nevertheless, increasing proportions of the new physicians will not enter the primary care specialties unless the residency mix is changed and/or the financing structure leans heavily toward reimbursement of primary over specialty care.

7. *Primary care practice will be offered increasingly in competitively advantageous organized groups.* Primary care is peculiarly sensitive to changes in (a) the overall array of residency positions offered, and (b) structural elements of medical practice. Structurally, the primary care function is likely to be most successful where there are organizational means to support it: through organized primary care practices such as family practice centers, through primary care insurance (such as SAFECO), and through HMOs which emphasize primary care. There will be an increasing number of organized primary care practices, such as family practices, primary care partnerships or clinics.

Aiken and others have pointed out that physicians in different specialties engage in primary care as well as specialty care,[3] but there is no simple way of measuring such developments. Specialists will undoubtedly provide primary care as an extended aspect of their practice. However, in an increasingly tight market, physicians in organized groups emphasizing primary care will have a competitive edge in terms of attracting and monopolizing patients. I do not see a huge potential for part-time primary care by specialists who advertise their skills in other fields. More probable is the formation of a primary care or comprehensive practice by a group of specialists who will be able to adjust their roles (and labels) according to their patient population.

8. *New specialty fields will be created but are unlikely to have a major impact on the total array of specialty care.* New fields worth mentioning are sports medicine, already well developed; vascular surgery, approved for a certificate of special competence by the American Board of Medical Specialties; nutrition, for which such a certificate is being sought; critical care, an area of potential turf wars within internal medicine and between internal medicine and anesthesiology; clinical pharmacology, hailed in the journals as a new speci-

alty; medical genetics, for which an "unofficial" certifying board exists; and clinical hypnosis.

9. *Specialties deemed by GMENAC as shortage fields in 1990 will continue to be in short supply.* GMENAC surmised shortages by 1990 in child psychiatry, emergency medicine, preventive medicine, general psychiatry, and physical medicine and rehabilitation. Except for psychiatry, the development of these fields is largely dependent on structural support, e.g., the development of hospital and freestanding emergency rooms, employment positions in preventive medicine in industry or public health, or the availability of funds for rehabilitation clinics. Large increases in third-party coverage for psychiatry are not foreseen. Residency training positions are not being dramatically increased in these areas.

10. *The medical profession at large will remain psychophobic and, with certain exceptions, uninterested in preventive medicine and rehabilitation, regardless of predictions of the "need" for specialists in several neglected areas.* Areas regarded as neglected include child abuse, drugs and alcohol, geriatrics, human sexuality, and nutrition. Presumably such skills would come out of general internal medicine, general pediatrics, and general psychiatry. There is as yet little evidence of interest in these fields, despite some optimism in the medical literature.[4]

Moreover, all such fields assume structural support, such as the development of clinics and established medical centers or public health programs. Some physicians may be able to make a living through freestanding practices, specializing in, for example, human sexuality, but any such development is likely to be at the margin of specialization as a whole.

11. *Specialty choice will continue to be strongly influenced by the perceived prestige of different fields, as reflected in the values and cultures of the medical schools.* Major changes in specialty distribution would require changes not only in residency education and in fiscal incentives, but in specialty status and in psychological attitudes within the medical field. Despite some promising examples, present trends suggest a narrowing, rather than a broadening, of interests and increased competition for traditional fields, rather than a widening of interest over medicine as a whole. (I should like to be proved wrong over this.) Critics have claimed that in the first year of some residency programs (surgery, pediatrics, obstetrics-gynecology, psychiatry, and pathology) knowledge and skills in broad areas of medicine are not sufficiently emphasized.[5] Geriatrics continues to have low status, as does the general area of nutrition and diet control.

The normative stance of different physicians—and the effect of personal values on therapeutic choice—require increasing scrutiny. It has been claimed, for example, that the moral stance of the physician is an important determinant as to whether or not to relieve psychic stress through prescriptions for benzodiazepines. Therapeutic attitudes range from "pharmacologic

Calvinism" to"psychotropic hedonism."[6] Values and attitudes toward children, alcohol, old age, sex, personal behavior, or drugs (including therapeutic drugs) infuse existing and potentially important new medical specialties. Yet these attributes are usually ignored in research.

12. *An increasing supply of physicians will encourage variation in therapeutic choices by physicians in the same specialties.* If, indeed, personal values (and other aspects of professional judgment) lead to different, but equally plausible, treatment programs, we may see both more variation and more acknowledgment of such variation in the future. Second-opinion surveys in surgery suggest that differences of opinion do exist. The increasing supply of physicians coincides with a rethinking of medicine as an exact, reproducible set of procedures in which what is "necessary" can be clearly distinguished from what is "unnecessary." In the future some specialty practices may develop particular "styles" of practice based, for example, on the use or nonuse of drugs, on exercise or relaxation techniques, and on conservatism or intervention. More generally, we appear to be on the verge of major attitudinal questioning toward what is "scientific" in scientific medicine. Whatever may be the impact on individual specialties, this promises to be an exciting period.

13. *The potentially huge field of behavioral medicine will continue to develop outside of medicine.* Industrial interest and professionals who are not physicians are moving strongly into behavioral medicine. With the development of programs for smoking reduction, weight control, exercise, and tension reduction by major industrial concerns, such as Johnson and Johnson, and with the growth of lay organizations, such as Weight Watchers, much of the potential of behavioral medicine as a medical specialty has already been diverted away from medicine. Each week, for example, an estimated 40,000 persons receive behavioral treatment for obesity under lay auspices.

Behavior modification is already well on the way to being defined as *education*, rather than as treatment.[7] Research studies indicating that behavior modification by relatively untrained personnel may be at least as effective as traditional medical therapies only reinforce this trend.

Psychologists, also struggling for position in the medical marketplace, are increasingly likely to move into behavioral medical fields, and physicians will find it difficult to recapture elements of behavioral medicine in the future. Indeed, the move is well underway. Health psychology promises to be an increasingly important field, but in the field of psychology rather than in medicine. Interesting clashes may occur between psychologists and physicians in the future.

14. *If structural and economic conditions are supportive, medical specialties will prosper in areas that will require a mix of medical and managerial skills.* An increasing number of physicians will label themselves as geriatricians, although the total is likely to remain small. Such geriatricians will receive most support when they are working in established medical facilities, such as medical

schools or HMOs. An interesting field exists for specialists in nursing home care, the so-called gerontophiles,[8] where special skills are required not only in the biomedicine of geriatrics, but in all aspects of management of patients in long-term care.

In some other fields, too, specialties may show themselves as most successful where they develop appropriate management interests. Radiology imaging is likely to become increasingly available to surgeons and internists. Thus, unless radiologists become more involved in the radiological system as a whole, they may lose out in the inevitable competition of the future.

Surgery is another field in which specialists with the greatest managerial interests may be most successful at a time of increasing competition. If, indeed, 20 to 40 percent of surgical procedures can be performed on an outpatient basis, and if, indeed, the power structure of medical practice moves to organized groups of physicians outside of hospitals, surgeons who develop an ambulatory surgery practice in independent centers may find themselves ahead.[9] Freestanding physical medicine and rehabilitation services, including physical therapy, fall in the same category. So do freestanding emergency rooms.

I think there is a potential market for well-organized physical medicine, which could cover everything from exercise programs for the healthy to stress reduction and obesity clinics, to stroke clinics, and to more traditional forms of rehabilitation. Yet the figures do not suggest a cadre of specialists to develop such institutions in a big way. There were 492 residents in training in physical medicine and rehabilitation (PMR) in 1980, of whom 283 were Foreign Medical Graduates (FMGs). While many, perhaps most, FMGs are American citizens who will remain in the United States, this number is still relatively small to produce major changes in the field. (There are fewer residents in PMR than in neurological surgery.) Industry may be a major force for change through capitalizing the development of physical fitness (rather than pathology rehabilitation) clinics, with reimbursement coming from persons enrolled in preventive medical programs as well as from insurance and Medicare, but this effort is likely to be seen as educational rather than as medical (see point 13), that is, independent of a specialty of physical medicine.

15. *Overall, the proportion of physicians entering the primary specialties will decrease; an increased proportion will enter superspecialties, and there will be some development of new fields or combined fields* (points 6–13).

16. *An increasing number of specialists will lead to increasing competition for a practice niche.* Physician location consultants will gain in importance. Investor-owned medical systems will become more appealing to physicians because of their marketing and capitalizing ability.

17. *In the short-term, specialists will become geographically more dispersed.* This process appears to be underway already, at least for board-certified physicians.[10]

18. *In the longer run, the specialist will look for a "job" rather than for a "shortage area."* With increasing numbers of physicians competing against each other, HMOs and other organized specialist practice systems will become both more attractive and more monopolistic. It will be impossible for a specialist to establish a new practice in an urban or suburban area unless it is a recognized part of an existing practice network. Physicians graduating in the 1980s and 1990s will see (a) a prescribed number of specialty "slots" by virtue of the number of residencies offered in each specialty area, and (b) a limited array of "slots," represented in the opportunities listed by professional placement agencies, advertised in journals, or available in HMOs and other systems through formal and informal communication networks.

The fact that physicians are expected to carry an increasing burden of debt at graduation—an average of at least $50,000[11]—suggests a decreased willingness to take career risks. In all these respects, the physician's choice will decrease. Without debts, an increasing number of physicians might choose not to take residency training or not to practice clinical medicine. In that case, medical education would be similar to legal education, a career preparation for many different purposes rather than for practice alone. Changes in the financing of medical education should be viewed as an important aspect of physician manpower policymaking.

An increasing number of recent medical graduates or residents will choose not to enter clinical practice. One "specialty" of the future may, therefore, be the decision to avoid a traditional specialty. But the debt burden suggests that most physicians will not be able to afford low-paying careers. They will be pushed into high-return fields.

19. *The workplace of many specialists will change.* With an increasing number of qualified physicians entering the marketplace simultaneously with pressures to control costs and reduce the amount of hospital care, relatively more specialist care will be performed out of hospitals and relatively less in institutions. Since institutional care tends to be more expensive than noninstitutional care, the average income of specialists will decline faster than general trends might suggest. Competition between freestanding specialist services and hospitals will increase. Hospitals will find it difficult to stem the growth of outpatient surgery, freestanding emergency rooms, and other specialist practice centers.

20. *We may expect to see a more deliberate defense of specialist practice in the medical and general literature.* In a climate of increased competition and increased criticism of overspecialization and overtreatment, specialists will be forced to justify and defend expensive practices (see point 4). As competition increases, specialists will attempt to focus more on their specialty, rather than to provide more primary services for the specialty patients they treat. Thus, we may see increased attention to procedures such as caesarean sections, on grounds of quality of care and quality of life. Physicians will also become more involved in social policy, using quality of care as a goal.

Psychiatrists, for example, will demand better institutional care for patients and the reversal of deinstitutionalization policies, to some extent. Surgeons will push to raise the utilization rates of apparently deprived groups, e.g., black children and the elderly, who have lower rates of surgery than whites. Specialists will be less circumspect than at present about criticizing the practices of their competitors. Pediatricians and internists, who are estimated to order more laboratory tests than general practitioners and to prescribe fewer drugs,[12] will justify their practices on grounds of quality. Family practitioners will flood the journals with statements on the inadequacy of primary care given by specialists, and the importance of continuity and comprehensive care. Such criticism will be good for the practice of medicine—and good for patient education and treatment.

21. *Boundary disputes will occur between specialists and between primary care networks and specialists.* Disputes may be expected, inter alia, between family practice and pediatrics; among hospitals, clinicians, and radiologists over imaging; between internists with special training in nutrition and those without, over control of nutrition clinics; and between physicians in other areas where subspecialty training is claimed (e.g., between general surgery and vascular surgery).

22. *Specialty groups and societies will act in the classic professional manner at times of abundant professional supply, i.e., to raise educational standards and qualifications wherever possible, but simultaneous pressures will make the certification process more flexible.* The American Board of Medical Specialties (ABMS) will continue to be an important arbiter with respect to new specialties, but it will become increasingly vulnerable to criticism in the next ten to fifteen years. The idea of subspecialization is already breaking down in favor of demand for certificates of special competence in a given area. This kind of question will become increasingly common if and as special competence certificates are allowed in areas such as nutrition.

A loosening of specialist credentialing makes sense—if only so that the American Board may avoid being stuck with the onus of planning across all specialist fields (by virtue of the cumulative decisions of residency review committees and certification procedures) and being open to new legal suits and criticisms as being in restraint of trade. Two possible scenarios can be envisaged: (a) The board certification system will remain more or less the same. Board certification will be challenged increasingly by medical schools, by public agencies such as the Federal Trade Commission (FTC), and by individual physicians as imposing unfair restraints on the practice of medicine. (b) The certification and credentialing system will be loosened significantly to allow for a complex matrix of examinations across different specialties and fields, and the board system will become less of a licensing system and more a multifaceted testing agency. Under the latter possibility, residency programs are likely themselves to become more flexible. Option (b) appears both more likely and more desirable.

23. *Residency switching and games-playing will increase.* Medical students may hedge their bets by taking a first-year residency in their second choice of specialty, and then switching to their first choice when the opportunity arises. A considerable amount of specialty switching may occur during and after residency training in the next decades. Such switching will become easier if and as the requirements for certification and special competence become more flexible. Hospitals will try to counter this mobility by linking residents, where possible, to future practice opportunities. It will be more difficult to plan for the future supply of specialties by rationing first-year residency positions.

24. *As fourth-year medical students find, increasingly, that they cannot obtain a first-year residency in their first choice of specialty, unrest will grow among both students and residents.* House staff unions can be expected to take up questions of the number of residency positions as a matter of national policy. An estimated 75 percent of house staff stipends come from patient revenues. The apparent trend toward reduction in the total number of residencies suggests that cost-consciousness is growing among hospitals. Residency training will continue to be important to tertiary hospitals as a mark of quality of care and of affirming their status as teaching institutions. At the same time, community hospitals will have no motivation to expand their complement of residents, and contraction in the total number of positions may continue.

Outside the major teaching centers, hospitals may develop more flexible residency programs, if only to serve their own needs. With a lid on the total supply of residency positions and concern in hospitals about reimbursement levels, residency salaries are unlikely to rise. There may well be a crisis in the number of residency positions made available to new physicians within the next few years; i.e., too few residencies may be offered to accommodate the total graduating class of U.S. medical schools. Such an event would tend to favor the elite schools, would lead to cries for federal residency programs in selected specialties, and would of course impose hardships on individuals graduating with massive debts. Residency positions in the Veterans Administration (VA) hospitals and in the armed services will take on added importance for the total supply of specialties.

House staff unions will play an important role in pushing for decisions on the number and distribution of residency programs, on compensation, and on national programs to meet specific future needs.

25. *Medical schools will be forced to take a more aggressive stance on the number and distribution of residency programs and positions.* While medical schools may have no incentive to plan their residencies as single, university-wide programs, the major departments will push for increased authority over the length and content of training programs vis-à-vis the residency review committees and the boards.

In order to help medical students alleviate the burden of massive debts, some medical schools may develop combined programs that incorporate the fourth year of medical school into the postgraduate years. Some medical schools may offer their residents university degrees or certificates as an addition or alternative to specialty certification. Medical schools as a bloc, both individually and via the Association of American Medical Colleges (AAMC), will have an increasing voice in the specialist-training process. Conflicts between the residency review committees and medical schools or between the ABMS and medical schools are likely to be determined by medical school interests.

26. *Constrictions on biomedical research funding in medical schools will lead to an increasing differentiation of medical schools in terms of their emphasis.* For example, the top forty medical schools may continue to develop as first-rate biomedical research institutions; the middle forty be wracked by turmoil as they compete for a shrinking pie of research funds, often unsuccessfully; and the bottom forty may become trade schools.[13] (The last scenario may be too extreme.) Nevertheless, medical schools interested in being effective competitors for biomedical research funds also have an interest in superspecialist residency training.

In addition, because of the attachment of residency programs to medical schools, all schools will be increasingly involved in both demand and supply questions for residents; i.e., concern about the placement of their graduates and about the distribution and financial burden of residencies affiliated with the university. Residency placement will become an increasingly political process, in the sense of dependence on established medical school networks.

This scenario of medical schools competing with one another conflicts with that described in point 25. Together the two processes suggest an increasing role for medical schools in specialty determination and more variety in specialist education.

27. *At the same time, a climate of constricting resources will force medical schools generally to become more conservative.* Teaching programs in areas which are not deemed essential to the mission of the school will be cut. Past flirtations with programs in the humanities and social sciences will become history. The recent rapid growth of departments of general internal medicine may not continue. A recent study showed that ninety-five schools had general internal medicine divisions, but most of their faculty were nontenured.[14]

Professional organizations of internal medicine will push to maintain such efforts, but the great majority of teachers in internal medicine will remain subspecialists. Programs in geriatrics and new programs that link medical school departments with community institutions are unlikely to grow rapidly. Thus, the general culture of the medical school will, if anything, be more specialist-oriented in the 1990s than in the 1980s.

28. *Physicians in established specialist fields will resist encroachment by other health professions.* This may be especially notable in primary care (where independent practice by nurse practitioners will be resisted), in pediatrics and

obstetrics. The lines between physicians and pharmacists may be drawn more clearly. Physicians and dentists will continue to compete for monopoly of the head and neck. While physicians may not be able (or wish) to capture the specialties relating to behavioral medicine (point 13), organizations of psychiatrists will probably urge for a tightening of standards for clinical psychology and counseling services. There will probably be conflicts between physicians and social workers engaged in counseling. However, behavioral attitudes within medicine suggest that physicians will not attempt to fight social workers for control of social service agencies.

Within hospitals, physician-nurse conflicts may arise over questions of skill, compensation, and control. Some hospitals may wish to substitute RNs for residents. Nursing organizations and unions, meanwhile, will press for greater recognition and expanded functions for nurses. Problems of survival for many hospitals may, however, lead to a truce or no conflict, in the presence of a common outside threat. The most successful hospitals will be those in which medical and nursing staff work smoothly as a functioning unit.

29. *Competition among specialties may lead to new, multiprofessional alignments in selected specialist fields.* For example, attending staff and nursing staff and selected specialties may elect to provide both hospital and out-of-hospital care. One possible model is an organized group of physicians and specialist nurses (and others) to take responsibility for a medical or surgical service, for both inpatient and outpatient work. Hospice and home care groups are other possibilities. In this respect, the concept of a specialty would be redefined as a service that includes both physician and non-physician professionals.

30. *The increasing number of women entering and graduating from residency training will have little immediate effect on the array of medical specialties.* Women residents in 1980 were relatively strongly attracted to internal medicine (but not family practice), to pediatrics, and to psychiatry; more than half of all women residents were in these fields. Women were disproportionately represented in physical medicine and rehabilitation, in obstetrics, in public health, pediatrics, and psychiatry. The shifts of women into traditionally "male" specialties is still relatively recent, making prediction of longer-term trends difficult. Women are under represented in the surgical specialties and in neurology. In 1977 one-third of all specialties did not have women residents; now all specialties do. It is possible that, with a tightening of total residency positions, women may suffer from a male backlash and find it more difficult than men to enter the specialty of their first choice. There are still few female role models in senior positions in medical schools.[15] Nevertheless, women will be an important component of house staff unions and an increasingly important voice in medical associations. Whether some medical policy issues will be taken up politically by women physicians as "women's issues" remains to be seen.

Traditionally, women have tended to favor salaried or similar positions, and to concentrate in urban areas. My guess is that women physicians will show heterogeneous patterns of specialty choice, but that they will continue to be drawn disproportionately to internal medicine, pediatrics, and psychiatry, and over the years may have particular impact in the latter two specialties. If present proportions hold, women may also become a major voice in the development of physical medicine and rehabilitation services.

31. *Specialists will be increasingly dependent on informal associations and networks.* Belonging to a specialist group of one kind or another—whether as member of the attending staff of a prestigious hospital department, as member of an HMO referral system, or as member of a regional specialist association or an old boy network—will become essential. Women physicians may or may not be benefited by the network system. One possible (if limited) form of networking might be alliances between women physicians in selected specialties and other women professionals, including nurses.

32. *Major specialist associations will attempt to increase their authority.* Organizations such as the American College of Surgeons and the American College of Physicians will extend their interests to include all aspects of medicine. At the same time, new specialty interests will spawn new associations. The organizational culture of specialties thus promises to become more complex. National associations will spend more time discussing quality of care and sponsoring critical self-assessment studies and justification of activities in their fields. Overall, organizational activity will increase.

33. *The growth of specialization and specialties will benefit, in particular, patients with complex medical conditions.* Subspecialties will be built on additional knowledge, technique, and skills. Medical groups and health care institutions will be increasingly self-critical and on guard against charges of overtreatment. Precision in diagnosis and treatment will improve. The technological aspects of medicine will prosper, and ingenuity will be demonstrated in improving technical aspects of care at minimal cost. At the same time, much preventive medicine will be given outside the medical specialist system, and there will be a wider range of variation within given specialties.

The link between expanded physician supply and specialization is, in the last analysis, neither simple nor clear. But while past experience makes prediction a humbling experience, two unequivocal statements can be made. First, an increased number of physicians will accelerate already promising lines of development in the specialties, rather than lead to radical new developments. Second, obvious incentives will encourage specialists in the system to maximize their opportunities through a monopoly of training, patients, or facilities, or some combination of these. The conflicts of the future are likely to relate to the second point: the numbers, types, and content of training programs; the development of rival patient care networks; "encroachment" by other health professionals; and the position of the hospital vis-à-vis other freestanding institutions.

The idea of a "specialty" does, however, need to be reconsidered. As the above propositions have suggested, the definition of a medical specialty will be far more flexible in the future than in the recent past, when it tended to be equated with the titles of the various specialty boards. Specialties are likely to be associated much more clearly with jobs and self-labeling than with training, at least outside the tertiary medical centers. Thus, comments such as "I run a stress clinic" may become more important defining factors than whether the speaker is a certified psychiatrist or an internist. While major reorganization of the formal specialty-certifying system is unlikely, there promises to be increasing attention to the idea of special certificates of competence from specialty boards, from universities, or from other agencies, attesting to skills in a selected area, whether gained through long-term or short-term training. Arguments can be made for the existing specialty certifying boards to become both more powerful and less powerful—more powerful in the sense of controlling residency programs at a time of increasing demand for residency training, and less powerful as university medical schools and house staff groups become more willing to enter the fray. But whichever the direction, there promises to be an increasing focus on the role of employment as a defining mechanism for specialists, and on the informal (self-defining) system. While the formal professional categorization of specialties may not change dramatically in the next decades, there will be increasing variation in the labeling of specialist functions and in the range of practice within formal definitions. It will be an exciting period, as medical specialties become more openly self-critical and more flexible.

With such movements, the concept of primary care will also have to be revised. Primary care is a function rather than a specialty, but the phrase tends to be used as if it were the complement of specialism. In fact, the complement to primary care is secondary (or referral or consultative) care. The complement to specialism is generalism. In the past, specialties have been seen as fragments of medicine, rather than as a variety of approaches or "cuts" to medicine in its larger sense. In the future, with the exception of esoteric fields in tertiary medical centers, more and more specialists should be able and willing to generalize over a broad range of medicine from the base of their specific interests and skills. This is not the same as saying that specialists should practice primary care. A more fundamental movement is beginning to take place. Integration of knowledge, rather than its disaggregation, is the major challenge to medicine in the next decades. Flexibility among specialties and generalist views among specialists are the necessary corollaries for change.

Notes

1. Graduate Medical Education National Advisory Committee (GMENAC). 1980. *Report of the Graduate Medical Education National Advisory Committee to the Secretary. Volume 1. Summary Report.* Washington, D.C.: GPO.

2. Williams, D.C. 1981. Surgeons and Surgery in Rhode Island, 1970 and 1977. *New England Journal of Medicine* 305:1319–23.

3. Aiken, L., Lewis, C.E., Craig, J., et al. 1979. The Contribution of Specialists to the Delivery of Primary Care. A New Perspective. *New England Journal of Medicine* 300:1363–70.

4. Beeson, P.B. 1980. The Natural History of Medical Subspecialties. *Annals of Internal Medicine* 93:624–26.

5. Gonnella, J.S., and Veloski, J.J. 1982. The Impact of Early Specialization on the Clinical Competence of Residents. *New England Journal of Medicine* 306:275–77.

6. Rosenbaum, J.F. 1982. Current Concepts in Psychiatry—The Drug Treatment of Anxiety. *New England Journal of Medicine* 306:401–4.

7. Stunkard, A.J. 1979. Behavioral Medicine and Beyond: The Example of Obesity. In *Behavioral Medicine: Theory and Practice,* ed. O.F. Pomerleau and J.P. Brady, 279–98. Baltimore: Williams and Wilkins.

8. Schwartz, T.B. 1982. For Fun and Profit—How to Install a First-Rate Doctor in a Third-Rate Nursing Home. *New England Journal of Medicine* 306:743–44.

9. Detmer, D.E. 1981. Ambulatory Surgery. *New England Journal of Medicine* 305:1406–9.

10. Schwartz, W.B., Newhouse, J.P., Bennett, B.W., and Williams, A.P. 1980. The Changing Geographical Distribution of Board Certified Physicians. *New England Journal of Medicine* 303:1032–38.

11. Knapp, R.M., and Butler, P.W. 1979. Financing Graduate Medical Education. *New England Journal of Medicine* 301:749–55.

12. Fishbane, M., and Starfield, B. 1981. Child Health Care in the United States. A Comparison of Pediatricians and General Practitioners. *New England Journal of Medicine* 305:552–56.

13. Perry, D.R., Challoner, D.R., and Oberst, R.R. 1981. Research Advances and Resource Constraints: Dilemmas Facing Medical Education. *New England Journal of Medicine* 305:320–24.

14. Friedman, R.H., Pozen, J.T., Rosencrans, A.L., Eisenberg, J.M., and Gertman, P.M. 1982. General Internal Medicine Units in Academic Medical Centers: Their Emergence and Functions. *Annals of Internal Medicine* 96:233–38. Also editorial, 239–40.

15. Braslow, J.B., and Heins, M. 1981. Women in Medical Education: A Decade of Change. *New England Journal of Medicine* 304:1129–35.

References

American Journal of Medicine. 1981. Clinical Pharmacology a New Specialty. 70:221–22.

American Medical Association, Council on Medical Education. 1981. Summary Statistics on Graduate Medical Education in the United States. In *Directory of Approved Residencies* 57–65.

French, F.D. 1981. The Financial Indebtedness of Medical School Graduates. *New England Journal of Medicine* 304:563–65.

Ginzberg, E., Brann, E., Hiestand, D., and Ostow, M. 1981. The Expanding Physician Supply and Health Policy: The Clouded Outlook. *Milbank Memorial Fund Quarterly/Health and Society* 59:508–41.

Heilman, R.S. 1982. What's Wrong with Radiology. *New England Journal of Medicine* 306:477–79.

McLemore, T., and Koch, H. 1982. 1980 Summary: National Ambulatory Medical Care Survey. *Advance data.* Washington, D.C.: National Center for Health Statistics. 22 February.

Moore, F.D., and Lang, S.M. 1981. Board Certified Physicians in the United States. *New England Journal of Medicine* 304:1078–84.

Stevens, R.A. 1980. The Changing Idea of a Medical Specialty. *Transactions and Studies of the Coll. of Phys. of Phila.* 2:159–77.

7

Physicians and Hospitals: Implications of an Expanding Physician Supply

FRANK A. SLOAN

The number of physicians in the United States rose by almost 40 percent during the 1970s, and widely publicized forecasts show a projected increase nearly as large for the 1980s.[1] By contrast, population grew 11 percent in the 1970s,[2] and about the same rate of growth is predicted for the 1980s. Thus, physician supply has been and will continue to be on a growth trajectory three or four times that of population.[3] Such a wide discrepancy must have far-reaching implications for this nation's health system, both in the recent past and in the future. This chapter focuses on the effects of trends in physician supply on hospital care.

By any measure, the hospital industry is large and expanding. Tradition and official statistics fail to identify most payments accruing to physicians for work they perform in hospitals. No direct data are available to distinguish payments to physicians for hospital work from that at other sites. But by basing the hospital share of physician billings on the proportion of their total direct patient care hours that physicians spend in hospitals caring for patients (.37 for all doctors, .33 for medical specialists, .51 for surgical specialists),[4] it is reasonable to attribute at least 40 percent of physician gross revenue to work performed in hospitals.[5] This amounted to $18 billion in 1980, compared to the $100 billion spent on hospital care in that year.[6] The combined total of $118 billion represented more than one-half of all personal health care expenditures and 5 percent of Gross National Product. Not only is this a sizable level of spending, but recent data indicate that hospital cost inflation is, if anything, accelerating.[7]

It is often stated that the contribution of payments to physicians to the total health care bill greatly understates the importance of physician decisionmaking, which has considerable influence over spending for the entire gamut of health services,[8] particularly hospital care. Expenditures for

hospital care are also influenced by many other factors, such as changes in
the demographic mix of the population, technological advances, and the
regulatory environment. Ideally, one should assess the influence of physician
supply as part of a broader analysis that estimates the relative contributions
of a variety of factors to expenditure change;[9] however, this chapter will not
attempt such an ambitious undertaking. Its objective is first, to assess the
importance of an expanding physician supply and increased specialization as
determinants of hospital expenditure, and then, to judge what influence
these physician manpower changes had on the growth of hospital expenditures during the 1970s and are likely to have during the 1980s. Expenditure
increases reflect changes in the volume, complexity, and price of services provided. Part of this exercise will therefore deal with hospital utilization
responses to changes in physician supply.

The massive increase in supply also has important implications for physicians as individuals who rely on hospitals as a major source of income. In
view of the fact that growth in the number of hospitals and hospital beds will
continue to be negligible at best, in sharp contrast to the greatly expanding
number of physicians, will recent medical school graduates experience
increasing trouble in securing hospital privileges? Will physicians resort
more frequently to antitrust statutes to gain access to hospitals that have
denied them privileges? Will salaried practice and other contractual
arrangements that give the hospital greater control over physicians' practice
become more frequent in an environment in which doctors are more plenti-
ful relative to hospitals? Will hospitals increasingly set themselves up in competition with office-based practitioners as suppliers of ambulatory care? And,
conversely, will physicians create freestanding specialized ambulatory care
facilities as alternatives to hospitals? Will expanding supplies of physicians
and other health professionals mean increased competition among these
occupations for access to hospitals?

The next section examines pertinent trends in hospital and physician performance and physician supply, assesses empirical evidence on the contribution of physician supply and specialization to hospital utilization and expenditures, and examines the likely effects of expanding physician supply on
physician-hospital relationships.

Descriptive Evidence

The number of nonfederal short-term general hospitals remained virtually
constant during the 1970s, as shown in Table 7.1. At the same time, the
number of beds in such hospitals grew slowly—0.6 percent per year—
compared with an annual population growth of 1.0 percent and a rise of 3.3
percent in the number of nonfederal patient care physicians (other than

Table 7.1 Trends in Hospital Capacity, Expenditures and Utilization, and Physician Supply: The 1970s

	Annual percentage change[d]
Nonfederal, short-term general hospital	
Number of hospitals[a]	0.1
Beds[a]	0.6
Admissions[a]	2.1
Patient days[a]	1.2
Surgical procedures[e]	2.4
Outpatient visits[a]	4.4
Expense per adjusted admission (1980 dollars)[a]	3.7
Expense per adjusted patient day (1980 dollars)[a]	4.5
Nonfederal, patient care physicians[b] (other than residents)	
Total	3.3
General/family practice	0.7
Medical specialties	4.9
Surgical specialties	3.4
Other specialties	5.2
Nonfederal physicians[b]	
Full-time in hospital	5.8
Nonpatient care (teaching, research, administration, other)	4.5
Population[c]	1.0

Source: [a]American Hospital Association. 1981. Hospital Statistics, 1981 Edition.
[b]American Medical Association. 1970. Distribution of Physicians, Hospitals, and Beds in the U.S., 1969. Volume 1.
[c]U.S. Council of Economic Advisors. 1982. Economic Report of the President.

Note: [d]All annual percentage change estimates are for 1970-1980, with the exception of surgical procedures, which are for 1972-1980. Physician data are for 31 December 1969 and 31 December 1979, respectively. The hospital years generally end 30 September 1970 and 30 September 1980.
[e]To compare growth in surgical procedures with growth in population, it is necessary to have the annual percentage growth in population for 1972-1980, which was also 1.0.

house staff). By 1980, there were 47 physicians per community hospital, compared to 34 in 1970. As these figures imply, the rise in terms of doctors per bed, though somewhat less, is nevertheless substantial.

The annual rise in total real (relative to the Consumer Price Index—CPI) short-term general hospital expenditures of 6.2 percent per year during the 1970s is the result of increases in patient days and outpatient visits, which are frequently combined into "adjusted patient days," and expense per adjusted patient day. About three-quarters of the increase in expenditures is attributable to increased expense per adjusted patient day. Yearly growth in the number of patient days, 1.2 percent, barely exceeded the increase in U.S. population, 1.0 percent, and growth in admissions was only about 1 percent higher yet. There was a substantial rise in the number of outpatient clinic and emergency room visits to these hospitals, 4.4 percent annually. The number of surgical procedures rose 2.4 percent a year, but the surgical specialist supply increased faster, implying a reduction in operative work loads per surgeon. In 1979, almost one-half of all hospital admissions involved at least one surgical procedure.[10] The numbers of physicians working full time in hospitals and of nonpatient care physicians increased much faster than patient care physicians in general.

The annual number of visits per physician, both total and hospital, declined during the 1970s (Table 7.2). Overall, the decline in hospital visits was about the same as in total visits, although there were some differences in the rate of decrease by specialty. Combining information on the increase in the supply of patient care physicians (Table 7.1) with the estimated change in visits (Table 7.2), we see that total visits and hospital visits increased, respectively, 1.5 and 1.7 percent annually. These estimates are slightly higher than those based on Health Interview Surveys conducted by the National Center for Health Statistics (NCHS), which show about a 1.0 percent annual change.[11] (The NCHS figures do not include hospital visits.) Surveys of general/family practitioners, internists, and pediatricians, conducted by Mathematica Policy Research in 1975 and 1979, show about a 2 percent annual decline in hospital work load per physician, an even greater decrease than indicated for these specialties in Table 7.2.[12]

Over the same period, real gross income of physicians increased 0.6 percent per year, while real net income remained about constant. The rise in real gross income coupled with the decline in visits implies that either fees rose relative to the CPI and/or the nature of a visit changed. Increases in the physician fee component of the CPI were not sufficiently large to explain more than a minor part of the discrepancy between gross income and visit trends.[13]

Estimates of the percentage of patient care time that physicians in the various specialties spend in the hospital provide an indication of the degree to which each specialty is hospital-oriented. Physicians in non-hospital-

Table 7.2 Trends in Physician Visits and Income by Specialty: The 1970s

| | Total visits | | | Hospital visits | | | Gross income | | | Net income | | | Hospital hours as % of total patient care hours, 1980 |
| | | | Annual change | | | Annual change | | | Annual change | | | Annual change | |
	1970	1980	%	1970	1980	%	1970	1979	%	1970	1979	%	
All physicians	6,294	5,242	-1.8	1,819	1,549	-1.6	123.4	131.3	0.6	78.0	78.4	0.1	37.5
General practice	8,316	6,787	-2.0	1,457	1,274	-1.3	107.6	117.7	0.9	62.4	62.0	-0.1	25.4
Medical specialties													
Internal medicine	5,787	4,940	-1.6	1,723	1,864	0.8	122.0	128.7	0.5	75.3	76.2	0.1	38.2
Pediatrics	6,984	6,627	-0.5	948	850	-1.1	111.5	111.4	0.0	65.0	60.4	-0.7	22.6
Surgical specialties													
Obstetrics/Gyn.	6,374	5,370	-1.7	1,406	1,128	-2.2	139.8	158.8	2.3	88.0	91.8	0.4	34.6
Surgery	5,792	4,707	-2.1	1,887	1,701	-1.0	145.4	165.3	1.3	94.8	96.0	0.1	44.7
Other specialties													
Anesthesiology	2,231	1,902	-1.6	1,936	1,660	-1.5	94.6	117.7	2.2	73.7	91.4	2.2	71.0
Psychiatry	2,523	2,303	-0.9	1,003	768	-2.7	99.5	85.7	-1.5	74.6	62.6	-1.8	27.3

Note: Gross and net income are in thousands of 1979 dollars.

Source: American Medical Association. 1972 and 1981. Profile of Medical Practice. Chicago: American Medical Association.

oriented fields (general practice, pediatrics, and psychiatry) experienced decreases in real net income (Table 7.2). By contrast, physicians in the most hospital-oriented field, anesthesiology, fared the best. More comprehensive insurance coverage for physicians' services rendered in the hospital than in the office provides one plausible explanation of these divergent trends in doctors' earnings.[14]

The Role of Expanded Physician Supply in Hospital Cost Inflation:
A Summary of the Econometric Evidence

CONCEPTS

The notion that physician availability has some effect on hospital utilization and costliness is generally accepted. Regardless of which model of the medical marketplace one accepts, a larger number of physicians, other factors being constant, implies higher utilization of physicians' services.[15] According to one scenario, more doctors will mean lower patient "time prices" and therefore greater demand; in another view, a greater number of doctors means more doctor-induced demand.

Where the extra utilization will take place is another matter. Greater availability of physicians should mean greater availability of ambulatory care; this may lead to a decline in demand for inpatient care because more problems can be handled in physicians' offices and physicians face less pressure to economize on their own time. Yet the fact that more patients are seeing physicians more often may provide a stimulus to hospital inpatient care. This is especially true in the case of surgery. The vast majority of surgical procedures are performed in hospitals. For this reason, although the net effect of an expanding aggregate physician supply on total admissions is the result of the relative importance of two offsetting forces, more surgical specialists should mean more surgical admissions. Some of the increase in surgical admissions would involve patients who might otherwise have been treated medically, but the net effect on total admissions of an increase in surgical admissions is plausibly positive.

Another descriptor of physician mix is the proportion of physicians who are specialists. Given the technical nature of much of specialty training and the content of specialty practice, it has often been hypothesized that admissions per capita rise with growth in the proportion of doctors in the area who are specialists.[16] This single proportion is a crude indicator of an area's doctor mix, but it is the only measure that has seen widespread use in empirical studies of hospital utilization and costs.

One of the most important sources of variation in mean length of inpatient stay is case mix. The link between physician availability and length of stay partly depends on how the mix of admissions varies with availability; and on conceptual grounds alone, there is no way of knowing whether cases tend to become more or less serious in response to an increased number of physicians. As the physician supply increases, greater attention by physicians to hospitalized patients may lead to earlier discharges, on average, and may also allow many patients to be managed better on an ambulatory basis following the hospital stay. Both factors might lead to shorter stays in physician-dense areas.

The rapid growth of hospital outpatient and emergency room visits is often attributed to the physician "shortage."[17] Care is presumably provided in such settings either when office-based medical care is geographically inaccessible, or when many private practitioners refuse to treat Medicaid patients. Yet when there are more doctors in a community, it is likely a greater number will be available for full-time work in hospitals. This latter supply effect implies that more doctors will result in more hospital visits. Thus, as with many of the above utilization measures, conceptual arguments alone cannot determine whether increased doctor supply has a net positive or negative influence. The net direction of effect can only be determined by empirical analysis.

FINDINGS

A review of empirical studies that have been reported in the health economics literature to determine the contribution of increased physician supply and specialization to hospital utilization and expenditures reveals inconsistencies in methods as well as in findings. Therefore, a degree of judgment was required to arrive at the estimates of impact that are presented here. Some technical details are provided in the Appendix.

Several studies have assessed the role of aggregate physician supply as a determinant of patient admissions to hospitals and/or length of stay. The most plausible conclusion from these studies is that physician supply has *no* effect on admissions or on length of inpatient stays.[18]

In 1970, 26 percent of patient care physicians were general/family practitioners;[19] by the end of the decade, they had declined to 20 percent of the total. From studies that have considered the role of specialization, there is a definite increase in both admissions and length of stay as the proportion of physicians who are general practitioners decreases. In quantitative terms, these studies imply that the decline of general/family physicians during the 1970s resulted in an increase both in admissions and mean stay of about 0.4 percent annually. Combining these estimates with the "best" (mid-range) estimates that aggregate physician supply has a zero effect, it appears that changes in physician supply and specialty composition together raised inpatient days some 0.8 percent annually over the level that would have prevailed had the number and mix of doctors (general/family practitioners versus specialists) not changed during the 1970s.

Studies of surgical utilization have focused on the effect of surgeon supply on the number of surgical procedures. Results of these studies suggest that the 3.4 percent annual increase in surgeon supply accounted for a 0.5 percent annual increase in the number of operations, about one-seventh of the total increase in surgical procedures during the 1970s. Estimates from a study by Fuchs imply that the expanding surgeon supply accounted for as much as one-third of the growth in volume of surgery performed.[20]

Unfortunately, no one has carried the analysis of effects of expanding surgeon supply one step further. Given that greater supply boosts the number of operative procedures, what happens to hospital admissions overall? In the absence of studies on the issue, it is still useful to consider effects under alternative (assumed) scenarios. Suppose that admissions rise 0.1 percent for every 1 percent increase in operations (low estimate), and, alternatively, every 1 percent increase in operations yields a 0.5 percent increase in admissions (high estimate). Then, according to the first scenario, the rise in the number of surgical specialists during the 1970s would have raised total admissions by a negligible amount, 0.05 percent annually. According to the second, the rise would have been five times higher but, nevertheless, only 0.25 percent. Thus, it is not likely that the growth in supply of surgeons during the 1970s had an appreciable effect on total admissions to community hospitals between 1970 and 1980.

Judging from the available studies, physician supply makes a substantial contribution to utilization of hospital outpatient care. A mid-range estimate from the more reliable studies implies that such visits rise about 0.4 percent for every 1 percent rise in physicians. (The estimates range from a low response of 0.3 percent to a high of 0.5.) Assuming a rate of 0.4 percent, about one-third of the increase in outpatient activity during the 1970s can be explained by the change in this one variable.[21]

To the extent that changes in supply and mix affect complexity rather than volume of hospital services, analysis of the above utilization measures may understate the actual influence of physician manpower changes. For example, it is known that there have been substantial changes in the mix of operative procedures and also dramatic growth in the number of ancillary services provided by hospitals.[22] Although far from perfect, hospital expense per adjusted patient day and per admission partly reflect changes in complexity. Studies indicate that expanding aggregate supply raised cost per adjusted patient day and cost per adjusted admission about 0.2 percent annually during the 1970s. The decline in the proportion of general/family practitioners raised real expenditures for hospital care by another 0.1 percent per annum.

Combining estimates of the influence of physician supply and composition on patient days and outpatient visits with their counterparts for expense per adjusted patient day, it appears that changing supply and specialty mix generated about a 1.25 percent annual increase in the nation's real spending for-care in nonfederal short-term general (or, equivalently, community) hospitals during the 1970s. In other words, if the number of patient care physicians and the proportion of general/family practitioners were the same in 1980 as in 1970, the 1970–1980 increase in real payments to such hospitals would have been 20 percent lower, and the nation would have spent $70 billion on care in these hospitals in 1980, rather than $77 billion.[23] Of course, any estimate of this type is subject to some uncertainty. Nevertheless, judging from the statistical evidence accumulated to date, changes in physician supply and composition increased real spending on care in community hospitals between 0.8 and 1.6 percent per year, for a range of $4 to $9 billion, with $7 billion as the "best estimate."

Relationships Between Physicians and Hospitals

Evidence regarding physician-hospital relationships is, unfortunately, largely anecdotal. With the exception of the Survey of Medical Staff Organization conducted by the American Hospital Association in 1972–1973, few studies have dealt explicitly with the subject, and data available from other sources are indeed fragmentary.[24] Much of the most recent writing is unduly pessimistic about the future of medical practice during the next ten years or so,[25] in sharp contrast to perceptions expressed several years ago that viewed the environment as extremely favorable to doctors. Even discounting for such fads, the environment in which doctors practice is changing. Although the hospital was once the "physician's workshop,"[26] this has become less true for a variety of reasons. I shall focus here on the role of expanding physician supply.

An enlarged physician supply has begun to have discernible effects on physician/hospital relationships. First, hospitals are finding more doctors available for full-time and part-time work as salaried employees.[27] Part-timers include those who want to supplement their earnings from office-based practice, as well as those who do not seek full-time employment in any setting, such as some female physicians in the child-bearing, child-rearing years. Increased physician employment is enabling hospitals to expand their outpatient service capacity[28] and to extend their offerings into new areas, for example, obesity clinics and cancer self-examination programs.[29] The latter specialized programs have in some cases provided a mechanism for attracting patients to the hospital for other types of ambulatory care.[30] From the hospital's standpoint, a degree of diversification may be advantageous because of uncertainties about the future of third-party reimbursement practices for inpatient care. In a few instances, hospitals and single groups of physicians have formed corporate entities for the provision of hospital and physicians' services.[31] Such horizontal mergers give the hospital greater control over its destiny and, at the same time, offer participating physicians a more secure level of earnings.

A second consequence follows directly from the first. There appear to be increasing pressures, largely from established physicians, for closed hospital staffing.[32] Since physicians who have resorted to antitrust suits to gain hospital admitting privileges have been notoriously unsuccessful,[33] such litigation may soon decline, even in the face of increasing barriers to hospital access.[34] The courts have recognized that closed staffing, even in the form of exclusive dealing contracts, has an economic rationale, particularly in specialized technological areas, such as pathology and radiology, where such contracts may improve coordination within the hospital, assure coverage and, in some instances, enable the hospital to realize scale economies.[35] But closed staffing also provides obvious protection for established doctors. There is strong evidence that it is becoming more difficult for physicians to secure admitting privileges at some hospitals.

Third, partly in response to difficulties in obtaining hospital privileges, doctors are beginning to open freestanding surgicenters and emergicenters in direct competition with hospitals.[36] These "para-hospitals," which offer facilities and services traditionally located in hospitals, are increasingly being run by physician groups on an independent basis. Such arrangements seem to be growing because they offer price advantages for purchasers of care, freedom from such hospital regulatory programs as certificate-of-need, and a profitable investment for physicians.[37]

Fourth, physicians are showing greater willingness to work at smaller hospitals, a trend related to the diffusion of board certified specialists to small cities and towns.[38] As a consequence, large teaching hospitals are losing some patients who could formerly be treated only in these settings.[39]

Fifth, an expanding supply of doctors coupled with additional practitioners in other health occupations has begun to evoke more frequent and fierce conflicts among the health professions. Some of the conflict centers around hospital privileges. Osteopaths (in a few cases), new health professionals, such as nurse midwives, and chiropractors are becoming more aggressive in pursuing what they believe is their right of access to hospitals.[40] Physicians (allopaths versus osteopaths) have fought to protect their turf by blocking other professionals' access to hospitals and licensure.

Sixth, physicians are under increased pressure to join health maintenance organizations (HMOs).[41] In some cases, individual practice associations (IPAs) are being formed by physicians as a defensive response to prepaid group practice. By the early 1980s, 15 percent of all U.S. physicians had affiliations with some type of HMO.[42] The most noteworthy difference between the HMO and fee-for-service practice is found in their hospital admission rates.[43] Thus, to the extent that physicians are more willing to join HMOs, hospital utilization may be expected to fall. While there is some evidence that the HMO market share in an area affects the admitting practices of competing fee-for-service physicians,[44] the growth of HMOs to date has not been sufficient to exercise a major influence on national hospital utilization and cost trends.

Discussion and Conclusions

Econometric studies of hospital utilization and costs provide one basis for determining the contribution of the substantial increase in physician supply in the past two decades, as well as of marked changes in specialization, to hospital cost inflation. Given the methodological and data limitations of many of these studies, however, there is certainly a danger of pushing the estimates presented in this chapter (and the Appendix) too far. Nevertheless, they provide a useful starting point for discussion. To the author's knowledge, no one has previously assembled empirical findings from various studies for this purpose.

The estimate that changes in physician supply and increasing specialization were responsible for a 1.25 percent annual increase in real spending for hospital care during the 1970s can be disaggregated in several ways. First, higher real expenditures reflect higher utilization and higher expense per unit of output. Almost three-quarters of the rise in real expenditures between 1970 and 1980 is attributable to higher expense per adjusted patient day, rather than additional adjusted patient days. Physician supply and specialization made a larger contribution, however, to the annual increase of 1.25 percent through adjusted patient days (three-quarters) than through cost per adjusted patient day.

Second, the 1.25 percent annual increase can be divided into 1) the part attributable to the rise in the aggregate number of patient care physicians (30 percent) and 2) the part attributable to the decline in the fraction of physicians who are general/family practitioners (70 percent). The second variable provides only a first-order approximation of the changes in physician manpower mix that have been occurring, but this is the single specialty mix variable that has seen widespread use in past research. Clearly, where there are many specialists, there also tends to be a disproportionate number of "super-specialists" who, on average, are highly hospital-oriented. Similarly, where the physician-to-population ratio is high, a relatively large proportion of doctors practice in hospitals on a full-time basis, providing a stimulus to hospital use.

Furthermore, there may be interaction effects between supply and mix variables and other determinants of hospital utilization and costliness that have not been included by researchers to prevent overloading an already complicated analysis. For example, in an environment in which penetration of HMOs is comparatively easy, an increase in physician supply may have a different impact than in one lacking such alternative delivery systems. Growth of hospital outpatient visits in response to expanding physician supply may be different in a state with a mandatory rate-setting program for hospitals than in a less regulated jurisdiction.

The descriptive evidence reviewed in the earlier section revealed that although hospital utilization and costs have been rising, gross and net income of physicians have been fairly stable, and work loads per physician have been declining, both in total and for hospitalized patients. During the last half of the 1960s and the first half of the 1970s, opportunities for physicians appeared to be unlimited. More recently, a number of articles have been written by and for physicians that convey a sense of pessimism about physician practice in the future. Since physicians on average derive about two-fifths of their earnings (author's estimate) from work in hospitals and therefore have a professional stake in such institutions, it is not at all surprising that a number of articles have dealt with changing relationships between hospitals and physicians. Although such writing is useful for conveying a sense of emerging trends, both authors and readers should beware of over-generalization.

Barring major changes in federal statutes affecting third-party reimbursement and/or in judicial decisions, which in 1982 seem unlikely, relationships between hospitals and physicians will change very gradually. Although there will be more doctors in the 1980s than before, an increasing and aging population, higher real personal income, and technological progress will be translated into higher patient demand for medical care, both in and out of the hospital. During the 1980s (as opposed to the 1990s and beyond), pressures of the kinds described in the previous section are likely to be concentrated in major metropolitan areas where doctors are particularly numerous relative to patients, and younger doctors will feel these pressures most acutely. Doctors will still be able to earn a handsome living but, in some cases, both income and professional opportunities will become more circumscribed. This will be to the advantage of smaller communities and hospitals, organizers of alternative delivery systems, and freestanding clinics that compete directly with hospitals. An increased supply of doctors will, however, diminish the prospects of non-physician professionals who are seeking access to traditional health care facilities, especially hospitals. Physicians will surely fight harder to protect their turf.

Although they disagree on particulars, both the Graduate Medical Education National Advisory Committee (GMENAC) and the Health Resources

Administration (HRA) of the U.S. Department of Health and Human Services predict a further substantial increase in physician supply and a decrease in the relative number of general/family practitioners.[45] The mid-range parameters used for the historical analysis of the 1970s, together with an average of the GMENAC and HRA forecasts for 1990, yield the prediction that the 1980–1990 increase in aggregate physician supply and in specialization will make about the same percentage contribution to growth of real hospital expenditures in the 1980s as in the 1970s. Since many other factors underlie future increases in hospital expenditures, and major changes in legislative or judicial policy could have a pronounced effect on the supply estimates themselves, it does not follow that hospital cost inflation in the 1980s will be as bad as, or worse than, in the 1970s. Nonetheless, changes in physician supply and mix, already largely determined for the 1980s, will continue to contribute to the underlying hospitalcost inflation rate.

Appendix

Rather than rely on a single study which, no matter how competently executed, has some deficiencies (data, excluded variables, patient border-crossing problems, etc.), estimates of the effects of expanding physician supply and the trend toward greater specialization upon utilization and cost of hospital care have been derived from several existing studies. All are based on regression analysis, with the observational unit varying from the individual patient to an aggregate unit such as the state; in a few cases, the data base was a time series of state cross-sections.

Empirical research on determinants of hospital admissions and patient days has thus far failed to reveal a consistent effect of aggregate physician supply on these dependent variables.[46] In all the calculations presented in this chapter, physician supply has, therefore, been assumed to have a zero effect on inpatient use. Although there is some variation in the estimated effect of the proportion of general practitioners on these same hospital utilization variables, all studies indicate that a high ratio of general practitioners has a negative effect on the use of inpatient care.[47] Mid-range calculations are based on a -0.3 elasticity for the influence of the proportion of general practitioners on inpatient days, and for purposes of sensitivity analysis elasticities of -0.1 and -0.4 have been used for the low and high calculations, respectively.

The few studies that have examined the impact of physician availability conclude that more doctors mean more outpatient visits provided by hospitals. In fact, May's regression suggests an elasticity of 2.4![48] I have not used that estimate in my calculations since (a) it is unreasonably high, and (b) the R^2 on May's regression is 0.035, which indicates that May was unable to account for the most important determinants of outpatient visits. Eliminat-

ing that estimate, it is reasonable to conclude from the available literature
that the aggregate supply elasticity for outpatient visits is in the 0.3-0.5
range;[49] a value of 0.4 was used for the mid-range calculations, and 0.3 and
0.5 for low and high values in the sensitivity analysis. There is, unfortunately,
no adequate basis for gauging the effects of physician specialty or employment status on hospital outpatient use.

Several studies of hospital costs have included explanatory variables for
physician supply and a rough measure of specialty mix.[50] A mid-range estimate of the aggregate physician supply elasticity on hospital costs per
adjusted patient day from these studies is about 0.06, and for the proportion
of general practitioners, a value slightly less than this, about 0.04. These
values were used for the mid-range calculations, and values half and one-
and-one-half as large were used as low and high estimates, respectively, for
the sensitivity analysis.

Three recent econometric studies have assessed the influence of surgeon
supply on the number of operations performed. The highest estimate of
impact is the 0.3 elasticity of surgical operations with respect to surgeon supply obtained by Fuchs.[51] Pauly, like Fuchs, used data from the Health Interview Surveys (HIS) conducted by the U.S. National Center for Health Statistics;[52] but Pauly's observational unit was the individual patient rather than
the data aggregates for twenty-two regions used by Fuchs. Pauly obtained
more negative coefficients on his surgeon supply variables than positive ones.
On balance, Fuchs's results merit more confidence than Pauly's for at least
two reasons. First, it is quite possible that misspecification of the market area
specific to each patient is the main reason for Pauly's findings. Second, a zero
or negative surgeon supply elasticity makes little sense conceptually. Third,
although R^2s are often low with microdata, Pauly's surgery regressions uni-
formly have R^2s below 0.05, which is low even for microdata.

The third study, by Mitchell and Cromwell,[53] also used HIS data, but the
observational unit was the HIS Primary Sampling Unit. The investigation
found that, for operations overall, a 10 percent rise in surgeon supply raises
the number of surgical operations by 0.9 percent, yielding an elasticity of
0.09.

Notes

1. Graduate Medical Education National Advisory Committee (GMENAC). 1980. *Report of the Graduate Medical Education National Advisory Committee to the Secretary, Department of Health and Human Services. Volume 1, Summary Report.* Washington, D.C.: GPO; and Stambler, H.V. 1980. Comparisons of Physician Specialty Projections, November 28, Washington, D.C.: Department of Health and Human Services (internal document).

2. U.S. Council of Economic Advisors. 1982. *Economic Report of the President.* Washington, D.C.: GPO; U.S. Bureau of the Census. 1970 and 1980. *Census of Population.* Washington, D.C.: GPO.

3. U.S. Department of Commerce. 1980. *Statistical Abstract of the United States: 1980.* Washing-ton, D.C.: GPO.

4. The proportions for all doctors, medical specialists, and surgical specialists are derived, respectively, as follows: American Medical Association. 1981. *Profile of Medical Practice.* Chicago: American Medical Association; Kirchner, M. 1981. Non-surgical Practice: What's the Key to Higher Earnings? *Medical Economics* 58(4): 182–97; and Mattera, M.D. 1981. Those High-EarningSurgeons: Who's Faring Best? *Medical Economics* 58(2):188–97.

5. There is empirical evidence that doctors earn much more per hour in the hospital than in the office; therefore, the 40 percent figure may be conservative. See Burney, I.L., Schieber, G.J. Blaxall, M.O., and Gabel, J.R. 1979. Medicare and Medicaid Physician Payment Incentives. *Health Care Financing Review* 1(1):62–78.

6. Gibson, R.M., and Waldo, D.R. 1981. National Health Expenditures, 1980. *Health Care Financing Review* 3(1):1–54.

7. Rivlin, A.M. 1981. Statement before the Subcommittee on Health and the Environment, Committee on Energy and Commerce, U.S. House of Representatives, December 15, Washington, D.C.: Congressional Budget Office (mimeo).

8. Fuchs, V.R. 1974. *Who Shall Live?* New York: Basic Books.

9. Such an analysis has been performed by Sloan, F.A., and Schwartz, W.B. 1983. More Doctors: What Will They Cost? *Journal of the American Medical Association* 249(6):766–69.

10. Commission on Professional and Hospital Activities. 1980. *Length of Stay in PAS Hospitals, by Operation, United States, 1979.* Ann Arbor, MI.: Commission on Professional and Hospital Activities; and U.S. National Center for Health Statistics. 1981. *Utilization of Short-Stay Hospitals.* Series 13, No.60. Washington, D.C.: GPO.

11. U.S. National Center for Health Statistics. 1981.

12. Kehrer, B.H., and Sloan, F.A. 1982. *Patterns of Delivery of Primary Medical Care Services in the United States, 1975–79: Findings from the Physician Capacity Utilization Surveys.* Princeton, N.J.: Mathematica Policy Research.

13. U.S. Department of Commerce. 1980.

14. Dyckman, Z.Y. 1978. *A Study of Physicians' Fees.* Washington, D.C.: Council on Wage and Price Stability.

15. See Sloan, F.A., and Feldman, R. 1978. Monopolistic Elements in the Market for Physicians' Services. In *Competition in the Health Care Sector: Past, Present, and Future,* ed. Warren Greenberg, 45–120. Germantown, Md.: Aspen Systems; and Reinhardt, U.E. 1978. Comment. In *Competition in the Health Care Sector: Past, Present, and Future,* ed. Warren Greenberg, 121–48. Germantown, Md.: Aspen Systems.

16. Feldstein, M.S. 1971a. Hospital Cost Inflation: A Study of Nonprofit Price Dynamics. *American Economic Review* 61(5):853–72; and Feldstein, M.S. 1977. Quality Change and the Demand for Hospital Care. *Econometrica* 45(7):1681–1702.

17. Parker, A.W. 1974. The Dimensions of Primary Care: Blueprints for Change. In *Primary Care: Where Medicine Fails,* ed. Spyros Andreopoulos, 15–76. New York: John Wiley.

18. Weil, T.P. 1981. Do More Physicians Generate More Hospital Utilization? *Hospitals* 35(23):70–74.

19. American Medical Association. 1980. *Physician Distribution and Medical Licensure in the U.S., 1979.* Chicago: American Medical Association.

20. Fuchs, V.R. 1978. The Supply of Surgeons and the Demand for Operations. *Journal of Human Resources.* Supplement. 13:35–56.

21. These results are supported by logit and discriminant analysis studies of patient choice of practice location. See Sloan, F.A. 1978. The Demand for Physicians' Services in Alternative Practice Settings: A Multiple Logit Analysis. *Quarterly Review of Economics and Business* 18(Spring):41–61; and Sloan, F.A., and Bentkover, J.D. 1979. *Access to Ambulatory Care and the U.S. Economy.* Toronto: Lexington Books.

22. U.S. National Center for Health Statistics. Annual Hospital Discharge Surveys (unpublished data); and American Hospital Association. Monitrend. Chicago: American Hospital Association.

23. The $77 billion estimate is from American Hospital Association. 1981. *Hospital Statistics, 1981 Edition.* Chicago: American Hospital Association.

24. See Shortell, S.M., and Getzen, T.E. 1979. Measuring Hospital Medical Staff Organization Structure. *Health Services Research* 14(2):97–110; Sloan, F.A. 1980. The Internal Organization of Hospitals: A Descriptive Study. *Health Services Research* 15(3):203–30. Steinwald exam-

ined trends in relationships between hospitals and pathologists and radiologists. His results are quite interesting, but they are not generalizable to physicians as a whole because of changes in reimbursement arrangements affecting these specialties in particular. See Steinwald, B. 1980. Hospital-Based Physicians: Current Issues and Descriptive Evidence. *Health Care Financing Review* 2(1):63−76.

25. See Benton, C.D., Jr. 1981. Can We Compete for Patients and Still Live With Ourselves? *Medical Economics* 58(13):73−77; Berg, D.L., ed. 1982. 1990: Will Private Practice Be Worth the Hassle? *Medical Economics* 59(3):52−86; and Menken, M. 1981. The Coming Oversupply of Neurologists in the 1980s: Implications for Neurology and Primary Care. *Journal of the American Medical Association* 245(23):2401−3.

26. Pauly, M.V. 1980. *Doctors and Their Workshops.* Chicago: University of Chicago Press; and Pauly, M.V., and Redisch, M. 1973. The Not-for-Profit Hospital as a Physicians' Cooperative. *American Economic Review* 63(1):87−100.

27. Berg. 1982.

28. Berg. 1982.

29. See Roemer, M.I. 1981. *Ambulatory Health Services in America, Past, Present, and Future.* Rockville, Md.: Aspen Systems.

30. Berg. 1982.

31. Berg. 1982.

32. White, M.S., and Culbertson, R.A. 1981. The Oversupply of Physicians: Implications for Hospital Planning. *Hospital Progress* 62(2):28−31.

33. Berg. 1982; Davis, J. 1981. Health Professionals' Access to Hospitals: A Retrospective and Prospective Analysis. *Vanderbilt Law Review* 34(4)1161−1201; Ellis, B. 1982. Physicians Press for Staff Privileges as Competition Rises. *The Hospital Medical Staff* 11(1):11−15; and Robinson vs. Magovern. Federal Supplement 521:842−928.

34. Davis, J. 1981.

35. Blumstein, J.F., and Zubkoff, M. 1979. Public Choice in Health: Problems, Politics and Perspectives in Formulating National Health Policy. *Journal of Health Politics, Policy and Law* 4(3):382−413.

36. Berg. 1982.

37. Ellis. 1982; and Vraciu, R.A. 1982. The Health Care System—Evolving Investor-Owned Sector. Paper presented to *Health Care Financial Management in the 80s-Time of Transition,* March 26−27. Association of University Programs in Health Administration, Cleveland, Ohio.

38. Schwartz, W.B., Newhouse, J.P., Bennett, B., and Williams, A.P. 1980. The Changing Geographic Distribution of Board-Certified Physicians. *New England Journal of Medicine* 303(18):1032−38.

39. Menken. 1981.

40. Blackstone, E.A. 1977. The A.M.A. and the Osteopaths: A Study of the Power of Organized Medicine. *Antitrust Bulletin* 22(405):406−7; Latanich, T.S., and Schultheiss, P. 1982. Competition and Health Manpower Issues. In *Nursing in the 1980s: Crises, Opportunities, Challenges,* L. H. Aiken, ed., 419−47. Philadelphia: J.B. Lippincott; Solomon, L. 1980. Panel to Eye Trade Restraint of Midwives. *The Nashville Tennessean* November 23; and U.S. House of Representatives. 1980. *Hearings on Nurse Midwifery: Consumer's Freedom of Choice Before the Subcommittee on Oversight and Investigations of the House Committee on Interstate and Foreign Commerce.* Washington, D.C.: GPO.

41. Berg. 1982; Ellwood, P.M., Jr., and Ellwein, L.K. 1981. Physician Glut Will Force Hospitals to Look Outward. *Hospitals* 55(2):81−85; and Friedman, E. 1981. Doctor, the Patient Will See You Now. *Hospitals* 55(18):117−28.

42. Ellwood and Ellwein. 1981.

43. Luft, H.S. 1978. How Do Health Maintenance Organizations Achieve Their 'Savings'? *New England Journal of Medicine* 298(24):1336−43.

44. Goldberg, L.G., and Greenberg, W. 1980. The Competitive Response of Blue Cross to the Health Maintenance Organization. *Economic Inquiry* 18(1):55−681.

45. Graduate Medical Education National Advisory Committee (GMENAC). 1980; and Stambler. 1980.

46. Davis, K. 1981. Implications of an Expanding Supply of Physicians: Evidence from a Cross-sectional Analysis, May 14. Baltimore: Johns Hopkins University (mimeo); Davis, K., and

Russell, L.B. 1972. The Substitution of Hospital Outpatient Care for Inpatient Care. *Review of Economics and Statistics* 54(2):109–20; Feldstein, M.S. 1971b. Econometric Model of the Medicare System. *Quarterly Journal of Economics* 85(1):1–20; Feldstein. 1971b; Feldstein. 1977; May, J.J. 1975. Utilization of Health Services and the Availability of Resources. In *Equity in Health Services,* ed. R. Andersen, J.Kravits, and O. Anderson, 131–50. Cambridge, Ma.: Ballinger; Juba, D.A., and Sloan, F.A. 1981. Effects of Prospective Reimbursement Programs on Access to Health Services. Policy Analysis, Inc. and Vanderbilt University (mimeo); and Pauly. 1980.

47. Davis, K. 1981; Davis, K., and Russell. 1972; Feldstein. 1971a; and Feldstein. 1977.

48. May. 1975.

49. Davis, K., and Russell. 1972; and Juba and Sloan. 1981.

50. Becker, E.R., and Sloan, F.A. 1982. The Changing Structure of the U.S. Hospital Industry: Effects on Hospital Costs and Profits. Nashville, Tenn.: Vanderbilt University (mimeo); Davis, K. 1981; Salkever, D.S. 1972. A Microeconometric Study of Hospital Cost Inflation. *Journal of Political Economy* 80(6):1144–66; Sloan, F.A., and Steinwald, B. 1980. Effects of Regulation on Hospital Costs and Input Use. *Journal of Law and Economics* 23(April):81–109; and Sloan, F.A. 1981. Regulation and the Rising Cost of Hospital Care. *Review of Economics and Statistics* 63(4):479–87.

51. Fuchs. 1978.

52. Pauly. 1980.

53. Mitchell, J.B., and Jerry Cromwell. 1980. *Physician-Induced Demand for Surgical Operations* (Final Report, Grant No. 95-P-97245/2-01, Health Care Financing Administration). Boston: Center for Health Economics Research.

8

The Future Supply of Physicians: Directions for Policy

ELI GINZBERG

During the past several decades (1950–1980) a series of governmental and nongovernmental actions, taken to stimulate the nation's supply of physicians, resulted in a dramatic rise from about 140 to 200 practitioners per 100,000 population. Major actors in this expansion were state governments, the federal government (after 1963), the medical schools—old and new—that responded to the lure of easy dollars, and the much enlarged cohorts of college graduates who sought entry into the profession.

The supporting cast included the substantial inflow of graduates of foreign medical schools (FMGs) who peaked in the late 1960s and early 1970s, adding as many as 4,000 annually; more recently USFMGs, American citizens who attend schools abroad and then return to the United States to complete their training and enter practice; and the American public, who demanded easy access to physicians, a demand that was stimulated by increasing real incomes and the availability of insurance and government coverage for a high percentage of all bills for medical care.

All signs were "go" until the early 1970s when Dr. Charles Edwards, then Assistant Secretary for Health in the Nixon administration, questioned whether the long-assumed shortage of physicians, estimated at one time to be as high as 80,000, might not have ended, to be replaced by an emerging surplus. Within a few years, Congress, in its preamble to the Health Professions Educational Assistance Act of 1976 (PL94-484), officially declared that the shortage was ended and established the Graduate Medical Education National Advisory Committee (GMENAC) to undertake a comprehensive review of medical education (both undergraduate and graduate) from the standpoint of the nation's need for medical services. In September 1980, after a four-year effort, GMENAC reported that, in the absence of corrective actions directed at reducing future medical school enrollments, the country would face a surplus of 70,000 physicians in 1990 and more than double that figure in the year 2000.

Those who have looked closely at the figures have agreed that the ratio of physicians to population in 1990, irrespective of actions that may be initiated to reduce the future supply, will not be less than 240 per 100,000. The analysis that follows will focus on two issues: (1) Is it possible to discern clues in the current behavior of the key interests capable of influencing the future supply to suggest the direction and force of the actions they will undertake? (2) What are some of the public policy concerns that must be considered in assessing the merits of different types of intervention to alter the future supply?

A number of early signs can be readily identified. The federal government, with the executive branch in the lead, has been moving expeditiously to retreat from an activist role in the development of health manpower, including physicians. It has eliminated capitation for medical schools; it has reduced grant and loan support for medical students; it has cut back on the National Health Service Corps. In short, the federal government is extricating itself as rapidly as Congress will permit from the provision of financial support for medical education via the institutional route or via the student aid route. The single exception to this policy has been a reassessment of its efforts to strengthen Meharry, Howard, and Morehouse universities where a high proportion, about half, of all black physicians are trained.

Because funds for research and service as well as for educational programs arc uscd to finance medical education at both undergraduate and graduate levels, the clear intention of the administration to decelerate its expenditures for Medicare and Medicaid and the stabilization or decline in support for research constitute further pressures on the financial viability of the nation's medical schools. If the federal government proceeds with plans to curtail the medical operations of the Veterans Administration, this will add to the strain. Legislation and administrative changes aimed at encouraging prudent purchasing by state Medicaid programs and other measures directed to constraining the rise in Medicare and Medicaid reimbursements are further serious threats.

The evidence is unequivocal that the federal government, which for the better part of the 1960s and the 1970s took the lead to encourage the expansion of the physician supply, is now aggressively seeking to reduce its financial support, direct and indirect, for medical education. The only questions that remain are the speed and degree of its retrenchment and the adaptations of different medical schools to the waning federal support.

So far there have been only a few clues as to the responses of state legislators to the impending marked increase in the supply of physicians. Some states have been discouraged from proceeding with plans to open new schools. A few legislatures that "bought" seats for students in schools in neighboring states have begun to cut back. Budgetary proposals are underway in several state schools to curtail a modest number of places in next year's entering class.

But the states have surely not picked up and run with the GMENAC Report's recommendation of a 17 percent reduction in entering-class size of allopathic and osteopathic medical schools by 1984 relative to 1980–1981. There have been moves to increase tuition substantially in several state-supported schools, but the majority have made only modest adjustments. A few have reduced their appropriations for the entire system of higher education and have left it to the president of the state university to determine the distribution of the cuts between the medical school and the other divisions of the university. A few have curtailed their allocations for the medical school's principal teaching hospital. But again, as in the case of enrollments, the declines thus far have been spotty and minimal.

One development is clear. The states show no inclination to step into the breech and substitute their dollars for those withdrawn by the federal government. By maintaining relatively low tuition payments in their medical schools, however, they have taken much of the sting out of federal cutbacks, at least for those students who enroll in state-supported institutions.

If one postulates, as one must, that a great many states will be under substantial financial pressure until the economy returns to a higher level of growth, legislators will be receptive to suggestions for reducing their appropriations that do not adversely affect the welfare of their citizens. It is doubtful, however, that they will move early or vigorously to decrease enrollments in their medical schools, in part because substantial savings would be realized only if an entire school were closed. State medical schools will probably have to assume their proportionate share of reductions in appropriations for higher education, and these could lead to reductions in enrollments. But aggressive action for the direct purpose of reducing enrollments would probably not occur until the practitioners in the state persuaded the legislature that the market was oversupplied with physicians. And even such an effort might not lead to restrictive measures if the parents of students seeking to study medicine formed a coalition with communities where physician coverage was still shallow or nonexistent. In such a confrontation, the legislature might decide to do nothing—at least until the emergence of a surplus was apparent to most of the electorate.

There is no single or easy way to forecast the initiatives that medical schools will attempt in response to substantial reductions in federal funding and more moderate declines in state support. In fact, they are likely to take no initiatives, unless their financial situation were to worsen perceptibly. They will probably respond to a lower level of government support by seeking new and expanded sources of nongovernmental income: higher tuitions and expanded faculty practice plans are likely to hold the most attraction. But with tuition in many private schools at the $10,000 level or above, there is a limit, especially in a period of diminishing student loan funds, to further increases. Similarly, faculty practice plans, which in some institutions currently contribute one-third or more to total revenue, are not likely to yield a great deal extra before the cost in terms of faculty dissension outweighs the benefits.

There is no question that during the period of easy money, medical schools moved very far to raise the faculty/student ratio. In theory, and probably in fact, lowering the ratio through faculty attrition and tight control over new appointments might provide some relief. But with more than half of the faculty holding tenured positions at present, this approach also has limited potential for contributing to fiscal solvency and stability, surely in the near term.

In sum, these considerations suggest that most medical schools will be reluctant, on financial grounds, to take the initiative to reduce enrollments, because of the loss of revenue that such action would entail without corresponding achievable cutbacks in expenditures.

If the profession and the public were to agree that a surplus of physicians existed and was likely to increase, states with multiple medical schools might take the radical step of closing one or more units. Further, if private schools sustained repeated deficits which their parent universities were no longer able or willing to cover, there might be no alternative for the financially distressed medical school other than merger with another medical school or closure.

It was stipulated earlier that the enlarged number of qualified college graduates who sought admission to medical schools in the 1960s and 1970s proved a major force in turning the desired growth of the supply into a reality. Query: What is likely to happen to the applicant pool in the years ahead as tuition reaches a new high, loan funds become scarcer and more costly, and a demographic reversal reduces the size of the college cohort in the 1980s by approximately 15 percent?

The concatenation of these factors surely suggests that the applicant/acceptance ratio, which declined from a peak of 2.8:1.0 in the mid-1970s to its present level of 2.1:1.0, will drop below 2:1, conceivably to 1.5:1, by the end of the decade. With this drastic diminution in the applicant pool, a considerable number of state schools that currently accept few or no out-of-state students, as well as certain weaker private schools, would face considerable difficulty in securing the number of matriculants they desire from among qualified applicants. Were this to occur, total enrollments would probably decline, possibly by as much as 2,000 to 3,000.

Faced with such pressure some, probably many, schools might adjust their standards to accept more out-of-state applicants as well as applicants who today must go abroad for undergraduate medical training. Nor can the possibility be ruled out that sufficiently distressed U.S. medical schools might accept qualified candidates from abroad.

Possibly the most difficult parameter to assess is the extent to which changes in practice and earnings in the years ahead are likely to affect the decisions of college students with respect to the choice of medicine as a career. We know that the ease of establishing a practice and becoming a high earner within a few years of completing residency unquestionably encouraged the numbers seeking admission to medical school during the 1960s and the early 1970s. If young physicians, on completing residency training, encounter increasing difficulty in setting up a preferred type of practice, and if current and prospective earnings appear to be on a downward slope, the fall off in applications might be substantial, the more so because of the heavier debts that many future graduates will be forced to incur.

On the other hand, there is a sizable pool of middle- and higher-income families who will be able to finance a medical education for their children, and it is unlikely that the earnings from medicine will deteriorate rapidly relative to the earnings from other fields of professional endeavor. The safest forecast is that there will be some reduction in the pool of applicants as a consequence of a more competitive practice environment with declining real earnings.

Two additional considerations about the future supply of physicians need to be entered into the equation prior to assessing policy alternatives. The first relates to the profession's response to GMENAC's forecasts. For the most part, the response has been negative. Even the chairman of GMENAC, Dr. Alvin Tarlov, has been partly convinced by his critics. In a radio interview, broadcast in June 1982, he admitted that the denominator—a needs-modified estimate of future requirements—was insufficient to justify the conclusion of a surplus by 1990.

The second point relates to the hesitancy of most of the organized medical profession to take any public position recommending a cutback in the numbers admitted to U.S. medical schools. The American Medical Association was under severe attack for many decades because of its restrictive posture toward medical school enrollments in the depressed 1930s and is understandably reluctant to acknowledge that a surplus may be developing. Unless the membership forces the issue, the leadership will seek to avoid what it sees as a certain loser.

As of mid-1982, the constellation of forces line up on the policy front as follows. The federal government is well on the way to extricating itself from any direct involvement in the support of medical education; if the administration succeeds it will exert strong negative pressures on both medical schools and prospective medical students through cutbacks in appropriations, reimbursement formulas, and loan funds. The states have for the most part taken no action to replace disappearing federal dollars, nor are they likely to do so unless their tax revenues were to increase substantially. With the exception of a few states, however, there is little to suggest early action by the legislators to reduce enrollments in their state-supported schools.

Caught in an increasingly serious financial squeeze, medical schools have little room for maneuver. They will probably resist reducing the size of their classes because of the adverse effect of foregone tuition on their budget, committed as they are to so many professors in tenured positions.

The pool of applicants is almost certain to decline, possibly substantially, over the remainder of this decade; but when one takes into consideration the large number of USFMGs, it is unlikely that a dearth of applicants will force a reduction in class size, especially since faculties will be loath to adopt policies that will speed their own dislocation.

Finally, the critical reception of the findings of the GMENAC Report and the reluctance of most sectors of organized medicine to express an opinion on the prospective surplus of physicians, much less advocate policies to cut back on the future supply, leave the issue of policy very much in suspense. That may not be altogether the worst of all positions since it permits time to contribute to a solution. At present, neither the public nor the profession believes that any action, much less drastic action, is called for.

While only a few benighted neoclassical economists believe that the presence of more physicians means lower fees (what they overlook is higher total outlays), many informed observers expect the increasing supply to facilitate restructuring and innovation in the health care delivery system. They are also impressed with the contribution of an enlarged supply to the diffusion of physicians to outlying areas. In the face of these and still other putative gains, the call for early and vigorous action to reduce the prospective numbers appears premature.

But if we are to benefit from delaying action, we must closely monitor and assess events that may transpire in the interim. Only in this way can we determine whether national policy should remain neutral and rely on institutional adaptation or whether societal interventions should be initiated to assure that critical goals are not placed in jeopardy.

Those who see multiple advantages and few drawbacks to the large increase in physicians call attention to a number of positive consequences. They observe that it is always preferable in a democratic society, which places a high value on freedom of choice in career and work, not to delimit arbitrarily the numbers of qualified young people who may enter medical school. Now that our society has paid the costs involved in expanding the infrastructure from some 80 medical schools to 126, has equipped and staffed them and almost doubled their capacity, it should not cut back on the additional opportunities that this expansion has provided young people to choose medicine as a career. With perhaps 10,000 USFMGs, demand is still outstripping even the much expanded capacity.

Further, it would make little sense to reduce enrollments in U.S. medical schools at the same time that thousands of Americans are continuing to enroll in foreign medical schools where the level of training is on the whole distinctly inferior. The end result of such a policy would be to enlarge the number of less well trained physicians who would eventually practice in the U.S.

One important indicator of whether the future supply of physicians is outstripping the demand will be the numbers of American students who continue to seek admission to foreign medical schools. Were these numbers to drop substantially, if not precipitously, it would suggest that young people graduating from college have lowered their assessment of medicine as a career choice. In that event, medical schools in the U.S. might want to reconsider their admission policies with an eye to reducing enrollments.

One important objective of the commitment of the federal government to the expansion of medical education during the past two decades has been to increase the representation of minority students among medical school entrants, which, in the case of blacks, rose from around 2 percent to 6.5 percent. Recent years have seen some regression from the peak, but the proportion is still about 6 percent. While the factors determining the number of qualified blacks who apply to and are accepted by medical schools are many and complex (including family background, the quality of their undergraduate training in science, the availability of grant and loan funds, and the attractiveness of alternative careers), a shift in national policy from expansion to contraction of medical school enrollments would act as a deterrent to maintaining the present level of minority group admissions. To the extent that a reduction in medical school enrollments would have this effect—and it is difficult to imagine that it would not—there is one more reason for caution before deciding in favor of a policy of contraction.

Those who are engaged in developing new forms of health care delivery are almost unanimous in reporting that the last years have seen a marked easing in their recruitment of physicians. If such reconfigurations and innovations lead to more and better care at the same or lower costs, the additions to the physician supply can be viewed as a boon. But these new departures and the associated changes in health care markets must be monitored and evaluated to determine whether, in fact, these favorable results continue. It is conceivable that new delivery modes will develop, speeded by the enlarged inflow of physicians, but that the quantity and quality of the resulting health care may not be a clear-cut gain and that costs, instead of declining, advance. Intensified efforts by many providers, old and new, aimed at marketing new health care services could lead to marginal outputs such as cosmetic surgery, weight control clinics, or spas, all of which would increase total outlay without effecting significant improvements in the health and well-being of the American people.

Recent analyses have revealed a close correlation between the increasing number of physicians and the parallel diffusion of specialists to outlying areas, cities of 25,000 to 50,000, which for the most part has brought a higher level of health care to many millions of the nation's citizens. Continuing increases may result in physicians' having more time to listen to and be concerned with their patients. We know from survey data that a major source of dissatisfaction among many patients is their inability to communicate at any length with their physician during an office visit and the inadequacy of the information that they receive regarding their condition and the regimen that they are to follow. In this sense, a larger and less-harried group of providers may be able to provide a more satisfactory level of care.

It would be stacking the cards, however, if one did not take note of potentially dysfunctional consequences of such an enlarged supply of physicians. During the past two decades, the nation has trained sizable numbers of physician's assistants and nurse practitioners, most of whom have made a place for themselves in the evolving health care structure. There are more than a few signs on the horizon that physicians confronting difficulties in keeping their appointment books filled may seek, through various devices, to constrain the growth of such paraprofessionals. This, in fact, is a recommendation of GMENAC. In the face of repeated evidence that these paraprofessionals have made real contributions to the quality and efficiency of health care, an erosion of their position as a consequence of the increasing supply of physicians should not be accepted uncritically. Over the long term a society concerned about escalating health care costs must reassess alternative patterns of utilization. Such exercises will probably yield a strong rationale for encouraging rather than inhibiting the use of paraprofessionals, especially if new delivery systems favor large multi-specialty groups working in close association with primary care physicians.

If, in fact, the availability of a vastly increased supply of physicians is translated into more and better health care delivery at the same or lower cost, that would be an unequivocal social gain. But if many of the new services provided are of questionable value—and some may even prove injurious—and total costs continue to accelerate, then the increasing supply of physicians cannot be viewed as a boon.

On balance, it would appear that in mid-1982 it would be premature to initiate a new national policy with respect to physician supply, one aimed at curtailing future enrollments. But there are sufficient straws in the wind to justify continued monitoring of the increased numbers who will be entering the profession in the years ahead. If these increments contribute to improved access, new and efficient forms of delivery, and lower costs, the policy of watchful waiting could be continued. On the other hand, if many new marginal services are offered the public, if more and more resources are directed to marketing such services, and if the total costs of health care continue to mount, then indeed the issue of the future supply of physicians should be joined and early corrective actions taken to reduce the numbers admitted to medical school. Careful observation in the interim should make it easier to achieve consensus and to determine the best ways to cut back if such action is indicated. Balancing the interests of the public that pays the bill, of the profession that plays the key role in providing the services, and of the young people who will seek to enter medical school will not be easy. But the decision will be more confidently reached and the approach will command greater agreement if the trends have been carefully charted and their interpretation widely discussed. The determination of the future supply of physicians is so deeply intertwined with the public interest that it cannot be entrusted to any one sector—neither government, nor the medical profession, nor young people in search of a career.

Index

Contributors

Eli Ginzberg, Columbia University

Stuart H. Altman, The Heller Graduate School, Brandeis University

Karen Davis, Johns Hopkins University

Dale L. Hiestand, Columbia University

Frank A. Sloan, Vanderbilt University

Rosemary A. Stevens, University of Pennsylvania

August G. Swanson, M.D., Association of American Medical Colleges